BEES HELP

FIGHT

VIRUSES

HOW TO PREVENT AND HEAL FLU,

COLD, STOMACH PAIN AND OTHER BACTERIAL

& VIRAL INFECTIONS

WITH HONEY, PROPOLIS AND BEE VENOM

by Mihaly Hevesi

Revised and Expanded Edition

Published by M&H Publishing V/Sz

Copyright © M. Hevesi
Published by M&H Publishing, 2020, 2021 Vienna/Szeged
Cover design by Healer Bees
ISBN: 9798651958375

FOR ORDERING INFORMATION OR SPECIAL DISCOUNTS
FOR BULK PURCHASES (RESELLERS, BEEKEEPERS, ETC)
PLEASE CONTACT:
hevesim@yahoo.com
www.healerbees.com

To my grandfather Mihaly and to my son Marcell

TABLE OF CONTENTS

TABLE OF CONTENTS

TABLE OF CONTENTS

TABLE OF CONTENTS

TABLE OF CONTENTS

Acknowledgements:

First and foremost I would like to thank my grandfather, Mihaly who introduced me to the mysteries of bees in a very safe and playful way when I was only a few years old. By telling me beautiful tales about bees and later on, when I was an adolescent, he showed me how bees can help with honey, propolis and even with stings during difficult times.

I cannot express enough gratefulness to my beekeeper and journalist colleagues for their continued support, encouragement and critiques along the way: José-Miguel de Santos, Peter Bross, Janos R. Kormendy, Matthias Winter.

I'm thankful to my wife, Eva, who has always supported me in my sometimes strange and out-of-the-box projects, like curing myself with bee venom. Without her help, I couldn't have written this book.

My special thanks go to Jennifer Tusz and Jeremy Parrott who edited the English for this book.

Last but not least, I'd like to thank the kind readers who have read this book and try to understand why bees help, not only fight viruses but in many other aspects of our lives!

Introduction

The message of this book is actually that by using bee products, you are able to get rid of invasive pathogens at the very beginning of an infection. Honey and propolis tincture, administered correctly, are able to destroy cell membranes of the pathogens in our mucosa. Thus, they can play a very important role in prevention. If pathogens enter at a deeper level, bee venom can help our immune system to fight the pathogens and in some cases it is able to kill these pathogens.

I'll share how I use these bee products to best deal with influenza, cold, and some gastrointestinal diseases, like peptic ulcers and other bacterial, fungal and viral infections.

The title of this book may be provoking, but there is valid scientific proof that the compound of bee venom, called melittin can destroy the HIV-virus, Hepatitis-B- and C viruses and it can kill tumor cells.

Another fact is that beekeepers exposed to bee stings have increased levels of IL10 (an anti-inflammatory cytokine). It is no accident that some medical doctors have proposed bee venom and propolis in the recent pandemic. Will this proposal stand up to scientific scrutiny? You'll also read about the science behind this suggestion.

During epidemics and pandemics health systems seem to be fragile. Unfortunately, epidemics and pandemics aren't black swans anymore (the "black swan" is a term used by Nassim Taleb for unexpected events) and due to the highly developed connectivity in our world, they will continue to occur more often than they used to.

That's one of the reasons why it's so urgent to know how to use alternative therapies that can help effectively.

In my opinion these high value materials – honey, propolis, bee venom (melittin) – should be used in clinics and not only in alternative therapies. Just as happened with Vivamel and MediHoney (both used in wound treatment).

Some developers/researchers are trying to capitalize on bee venom or its synthetic variants right now. I truly hope they'll succeed.

I also hope that this book will help you appreciate and admire bees not only for their indispensable work in pollination, but also for their amazing life and products which can help to maintain and improve our health.

This book is for informational purposes only and it is not a substitute for medical advice, diagnosis or treatment. Consult your physician whenever you plan to make substantial changes in your diet or therapies. If you have any medical issues always consult your doctor first. (Please read also the Medical Disclaimer at the end of this book!)

About myself and this book

I'm a beekeeping journalist, third generation beekeeper and teacher aiming to share my nearly four decades of personal self-healing experience and knowledge about bees and bee products.

Although I am a bee enthusiast and I've been keeping bees since childhood, I am serious about not giving untested information here.

I'll stick to the facts and, of course, I'll let you know about the disadvantages as well.

What will you learn from this book?

As the title of this book promises prevention of common infections (cold, flu, gastritis), I will go into some details of the nature of infections, and how we can reduce them in our bodies.

You'll also read about some known and less known hygienic measures like throat, mouth and sinus cleaning, and some lifestyle changes which are important for the prevention of many infectious diseases.

I'll describe then primarily three bee products that have helped me with health issues.

One is commonly known: it is honey. You'll learn why the smart and regular consumption of honey in the morning and at bedtime is the best choice for achieving an overall healthy physical condition or for protecting and reestablishing the balance of gut microbiota ecosystem, reducing high cholesterol levels, in some cases also obesity, getting rid of insomnia, improving blood sugar levels and boosting our immune system.

You'll learn how to use honey, which honey variety to use and when it is better to avoid it.

Another bee product is propolis, which is less well-known but is a powerful remedy in fighting and preventing viral, bacterial and fungal infections. It appears to be a very effective natural remedy against different ulcers and in healing injuries and cuts.

I'll describe how I had healed my gastric ulcer with propolis. You'll be taught how you can prepare your own propolis tincture.

I think the most important and interesting part of this book is the bee venom cure I applied to myself and which helped me when an aggravated flu sent me to bed for several weeks with a coughing attack.

When using bee venom, precaution is needed, but for those suffering from long-lasting and chronic conditions, like Lyme-disease, multiple sclerosis, arthritis and other autoimmune diseases, it can be a viable consideration if controlled by an expert.

You'll also learn about success stories that confirm that bee venom is an effective additive therapy for the above diseases. But you'll be warned about the dangers of such therapies as well.

I'll also describe how I keep bees – besides in my apiary – in an observation hive that I use for educational purposes and for self-healing.

I am republishing in this book an interview I made for beekeeping journals with leading apitherapist Dr. Stefan Stangaciu. The interview reveals important information about our immune systems and about bee products, including practical and technical information about their application.

When the use of bee products is combined with proper hygiene and some lifestyle choices – checking what diet is right for you or improving your sleeping pattern –, the effects won't be only transient but lasting ones.

You'll read about how to make life style changes by "knowing yourself" at the end of the book. Experiencing what is good for you can help you tailor an individual lifestyle change both for your health and a fulfilled life.

I wish you a healthy life and a nice journey through the world of bee products and simple self-healing techniques this book is intended to provide!

1. PREVENTION BY HYGIENE AND THE NATURE OF INFECTIONS

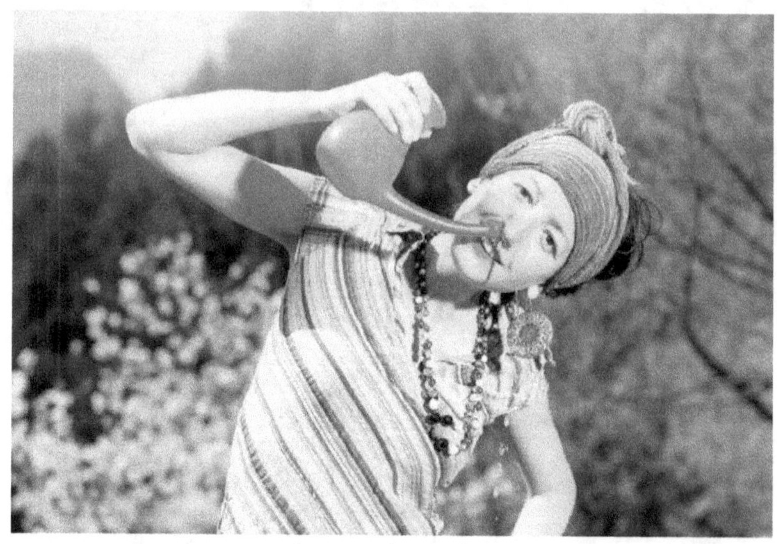

In this section you'll learn:

- The use of some simple hygienic measures;

- Why good bacteria are important for our health;

- What inflammation is and how we get infections;

- The good news: we can recognize when we are exposed to pathogens;

A doctor substitute: one of my basic "flu experiences"

Unfortunately, I used to be susceptible to different infectious diseases. When I was a child and caught a cold my mom used to give me an anti-pyretic suppository to reduce my fever.

That was probably a great mistake, as nowadays fever is acknowledged as one of our body's self-healing powers and many physicians no longer advise reducing it unless it's very high.

If the suppository failed to reduce my fever, my mom took me to the doctor to get antibiotics. In most cases, I recovered more or less in a few days or in a week, probably due to my young immune system.

The first time I experienced a longer lasting cold was in my twenties when I was a college student. Though I got some antibiotics – because the doctor I visited thought it was a bacterial infection (antibiotics don't work against viruses!) – I failed to recover in a few days. Even after two weeks I wasn't able to attend courses and seminars, or to work at my student job. I still had to stay in bed, had a bad cough and a sore throat.

I returned to the doctor's in very bad shape. But this time I found his colleague, an older fellow about 75 who was very talkative. He had just stepped in for his younger colleague who had caught the flu. He said that he was a happy grandfather, spending most of his time caring for his two sweet grandchildren.

After examining me and thinking about my condition he advised me to quit taking the antibiotics and to gargle (3-5 times at once) with baking soda (Sodium bicarbonate) and some salt in a glass of water every half hour.

I was astonished because I expected some drugs or another antibiotic, but I followed his advice and my sore throat was gone by the next morning and I was able to return to work by the second day. One may say the illness had already come to its end, the gargling only washed out and gave a last blow to the already weakened pathogens in my throat. That would probably be right.

Even now, when following the pandemic news, one of the medical findings is that the virus stays in the throat for days before attacking the lungs and spreading in our body. Of course gargling with baking soda isn't enough against a virus, but it is a good measure to reduce its numbers! If you add the correct consumption of honey and propolis to this preventive measure, you have a powerful tool in your hands against pathogens.

This observation is worth one or two thoughts.

> *Why isn't gargling part of our hygienic behavior to clean our throat, just like frequent hand washing (especially advised in pandemic periods)?*

Yes, we do some gargling when cleaning our teeth. But are we doing it in a profound way?

Try an experiment: drink or eat some chocolate in the morning and gargle in the evening or next morning. You will see that even after such a relatively long time, brownish bits will come from your throat. Isn't that the perfect terrain for pathogens to multiply?

If you don't experience this, you may have a lucky constitution or you may have favorable habits like drinking a lot of water/tea. But in most cases people are astonished to see these small brownish things coming out from their mouth even if they regularly brush their teeth but don't do profound gargling!

The issue of mouth hygiene comes to light in intensive care as well. When patients are put on ventilators some 15-45% of them get pneumonia! That is a serious issue in this area! The good news is that through a simple method it is possible to reduce the number of such infections: the assistants clean their patients' teeth three times a day and diminish the amount of bacteria being hosted in the mouth cavity.

The good news

An important aspect of most infections, especially respiratory ones causing Covid-19, flu, cold, or pneumonia, is that the pathogens first invade our mouth, sinuses, throat and upper respiratory tract. Before getting to deeper levels they actually stay on the surface in our mucosa for up to a week. The signs may be expectoration: runny nose, coughing up some phlegm, slight pressure in the upper chest, headache, diarrhea, fever, nausea, etc.[1]

When we realize that we are being attacked by pathogens, we should choose the best treatment: gargling with baking soda and salt, ingesting honey correctly (ingesting it very slowly and not eating or drinking afterwards for 30-60 minutes), ingesting vitamins (C, B, D), minerals (zinc, magnesium, calcium etc.), drinking enough water, inhaling honey and using propolis, having a sauna, fasting, washing through our sinuses and, if the invasion is advanced, using bee stings.

Nasal hygiene

Mouth, throat or nasal and sinus cavity hygiene seems to be important with infectious cold-related diseases and probably with other infectious diseases as well!

Actually, our sinus and nasal cavity is cleaning itself when we have a runny nose. We don't need to necessarily think it is flu or use drugs in this case.

It's believed that when we humans stood erect in the remote past our sinuses lost the body's favorable positions to clean themselves. This may be one of the reasons that pets or animals never catch colds. The self-cleaning ability of their sinuses still works very well.

The simplest way to rinse your sinuses is somewhat "disgusting". At least when I used to do it instinctively as a child, my mom wasn't too enthusiastic about that. I used to suck the mucus from my nose into my mouth and swallow or spit it. Well, my mom was probably right in suggesting to blow my nose and use a handkerchief. Sucking up mucus through your nose won't be appreciated by most people. But she wasn't right from a physiological point of view, because mucus can pass more easily through the "backdoor". Fine tuning this, you can press your nostrils alternately with your thumb or index finger and suck up the mucus, ouch, then spit it out or even swallow it. Of course only when no one is watching (i.e. in the bathroom).

Some children have a constant runny nose because of sinusitis that can drive parents crazy if doctors fail to cure it with common drugs or antibiotics.

Usually there is no need for drugs either. Again hygiene is the best! There are doctors, experts who can wash the sinuses with a special method.

If you or your child is troubled by a constant runny nose and you cannot rinse it correctly, find such specialists. After the cleaning sessions these experts do, the sinuses will be freed, for a while, from pathogens.

While not too often, but sometimes, when I am on holiday at the seaside I can also do something to wash my sinuses and nasal cavities "naturally" as well.

I swim a lot without snorkel and when diving I do somersaults and let the seawater get in my nasal cavities.

I admit, it's not a very pleasant feeling what comes next or to stay afterwards on the beach and let the water run out from my nose, but it's probably the best way to wash through my sinuses on my own.

How to do nasal irrigation?

A saline spray can clear out mucus and allergens from sinuses and the nose.

But if this doesn't work you can also use a pump designed for this purpose, or a pot with a long spout, called a neti pot. Using a neti pot is the most "pleasant" way, as due to gravity, the solution runs through your nose and it isn't pressed into it.

Use 1 teaspoon of non-iodized salt and half teaspoon of baking soda. Mix them in – 230-250 ml (8 US fl. oz.) of sterilized water. You can sterilize the mixture by boiling it for a few minutes and then let it cool down. Tap water is not good for rinsing your nasal cavities as it can contain contaminants. By the way, it is very important to properly clean your device you use for irrigation. It is best to use a non-plastic device that you can sterilize in boiling water for 5-10 minutes.

Fill the device with the solution you have prepared; lean over your bowl or sink. Standing in the shower is also a viable way to do the rinsing.

Incline your head sideways with your forehead and chin level. Breathing through your mouth, place the neti pot or container into your upper nostril and let the solution run into your nose. Then allow the water to drain out through the other nostril naturally.

Repeat this by turning your head the other way. You can do the whole procedure again and again until your nasal passages feel clearer.

If you can do it, turn your head in such a way that it is almost upside down in order to let the water get into the deep sinus passageways which are at the very top of the nasal cavity.

If you are unsure about using nasal irrigation, talk with your physician or find a specialist who can do it for you.

Bad bacteria vs good bacteria and antibiotics

Now let's look at why we should like the microorganisms and befriend the idea that most of them, even the bad ones (!) can actually be our friends rather than our enemies.

We live together with many bacteria. Moreover, they seem to constitute the basis of our health. Trillions of them are part of the microbiome ecosystem of our body in our intestines and different cavities, but they are also present on our skin, playing a protective role.

The good bacteria apparently regulate many of our body functions. When they are damaged we fall ill, depressed, can get other psychological illnesses or even die.

Meanwhile, the damaged microbiome had been associated with chronic diseases, such as obesity, diabetes mellitus, inflammatory bowel disease, alcoholic liver disease, nonalcoholic fatty liver disease, metabolic syndrome, atherosclerosis, cirrhosis, and hepatocellular carcinoma.[2]

The book *Gut: The Inside Story of Our Body's Most Underrated Organ* by Giulia Enders relates this in a very comprehensive and entertaining way and it's worth a read by anyone who'd like to understand the importance of the bacteria in our body.

That's why it is so important to care for our microbiome in any way possible. Bee products like honey and propolis are very effective at protecting and helping our microbiome.

Eating resistant starch and enough fibre can be a life saving measure. (See in *Take care of your digestive system,* page 31)

But there are bad bacteria as well, which invade and trigger infection in our body.

Since the beginning of the 20th century, different antibiotics have been the best choice to get rid of many of the bad bacteria.

But we have two issues with antibiotics. The first is that their use can cause bad bacteria to become resistant. That means during the "killing process" by the antibiotics, some bacteria – those which can't be destroyed by the antibiotics – survive and they'll reproduce. Researchers and physicians fear that in a few years some or many of the administered antibiotics will be useless in many countries. Not all countries will be affected to the same extent, as the use and administration is different. Unfortunately, due to very high costs, it's not profitable for pharmaceutical companies to develop new, secure and effective antibiotics.

The other issue with antibiotics is that, although they are moderately toxic in humans, they indiscriminately destroy bacteria, which means even good bacteria are killed. We don't exactly know what damage antibiotics cause in our gut microbiome over the long term, though it's sure that the advantages – killing bad bacteria –until now, have probably exceeded the drawbacks, as they helped to get rid of many lethal or long-lasting infectious diseases.

Viruses

Viruses are found in every ecosystem of our planet. They are the most frequent type of biological entity and are about a hundred times smaller than bacteria.

We are hosts to some viruses, too – like herpes virus – and when our immune system is down they can come to light. But in contrast to bacteria, there are no "good" viruses that help our health, at least not to our present knowledge.

Some of them may cause severe diseases in humans, some only in animals, plants or other living entities.

More than 200 viruses are acknowledged to cause human diseases.[3] The most known are: Epstein-Barr virus (EBV), hepatitis B (HBV) and C (HCV) viruses, human immunodeficiency virus (HIV), herpes simplex virus (HSV) , rabies and Ebola virus.

The WHO reported (in 2012) 1.5 million deaths caused by HIV, 80% of liver cancer deaths caused by hepatitis viruses, 400 million people living with hepatitis B or C, 500 thousand cases of cervical cancer caused by HPV infection.

One of the main differences between bacteria and viruses is that bacteria can multiply by dividing themselves when circumstances are favorable in their environment or in a host: first into two, then four, then eight etc., while viruses cannot divide on their own, they need a host.

When host cells are infected by a virus they are forced to produce thousands of copies of the virus. That's how viruses multiply.

Antibiotics don't work against viruses. That's why when patients with flu symptoms visit the doctor, he or she doesn't usually administer antibiotics. That also would contribute to making some bacteria resistant.

But researchers develop vaccines against viruses. Putting it in a very simplified way: our immune system is "trained" by being exposed to a weakened version of the virus. When we are exposed to and infected by this specific virus, later on our immune system is able to recognize it and act against it. Vaccines can be created from killed viruses or antigens: the viral proteins.

The use of vaccines has led to a dramatic drop in illnesses and mortality associated with viral infections, such as mumps and rubella, polio, and measles.[4] Smallpox infections have been practically eradicated by the use of vaccines.

Unfortunately vaccines cannot be developed against all viruses, (e.g HIV). There are only some drugs that can weaken their effects to a certain extent.

But there is another problem with viruses. As a researcher team reports from the Department of Physiological Sciences, University of Brasília: "Viruses exhibit rapid mutational capacity to trick and infect host cells, sometimes assisted through virus-coded peptides that counteract host cellular immune defense. Although a large number of compounds have been identified as inhibiting various viral infections and disease progression, it is urgent to achieve the discovery of more effective agents."[5]

The good news is that melittin in bee venom has been found to act against viruses. (See in *A promissing inovation, page 151*).

Trainers of our immune system?

Some scientists claim that these microorganisms can be seen as trainers of our immune system in a complex ecological environment.

The majority of malevolent microorganisms don't aim to kill us, as that would mean their death, too.

But if during such an invasion our body is overworked, weakened by stress, lack of sleep, malnutrition or poor nutrition, lack of movement, sun, or different macro- and microelements, we can suffer severely or even die.

Thus, bad microorganisms attack or invade our body, which causes infection and shows us that there is something that needs correction.

When treating ourselves, we must pay attention to all deficiencies and correct them and reduce chronic infections, if these are present in our body.

Infections and inflammations

Our immune system is normally able to fight the pathogens invading our body. But for different reasons it can become weakened or overwhelmed and doesn't accomplish its function of protecting us. The reasons for a malfunctioning immune system may be: lack of various proteins, minerals, vitamins, fats, carbohydrates in our diet; metabolic stress, leaky guts; lack of activity; lack of social contacts; insomnia; hidden diseases or too many invading viral or bacterial entities, which is to say in times of epidemics in our environment.

Inflammation is a protective process of the body. The body tries to regain balance by fighting through inflammation against the invaders or different existing conditions.

But on the other hand chronic inflammation can cause diseases like diabetes, cardiovascular disease, rheumatoid arthritis, obesity, liver inflammation, asthma, inflammatory bowel disease, Amyotrophic Lateral Sclerosis, Parkinson's disease etc.

Another problem when our immune system fights against invaders is that it can overreact. A so-called cytokine storm can be also damaging. But there are cytokines which regulate these overreactions.

Interestingly, beekeepers – when exposed to bee stings –have increased levels of these downregulating cytokines for some days (IL10).[6]

It is also interesting that the immune systems of insects, including bees, work in a different way to the human immune system. They don't have immune memory like humans have, and that is what is activated when we are vaccinated against viruses. Through our immune memory, our immune system will recognize and act against the once encountered virus.

In fact we don't know too much about the immune system of bees or insects and this is an area of the science where many things are waiting to be discovered.

But just as in the case of honey, which serves as a potential energy supply for the bees in the winter – it can be instantly absorbed and transformed by the bees into warmth – it's not impossible that bee venom serves the bees to fight pathogens in their environment or in their body in the most effective way. Bee venom is probably not only a poison to fight honey hunters and protect the colony, but also an important part of their immune system.

Summary

- We live together with many bacteria. Trillions of them are part of our microbiome ecosystem of our body.

- Good bacteria apparently regulate some of our body functions.

- The damaged microbiome had been associated with some chronic diseases,

- We are hosts to some viruses, too- like herpes virus – and when our immune system is down they can come to light.

- More than 200 viruses are acknowledged to cause human diseases like hepatitis B (HBV) and C (HCV) viruses, human immunodeficiency virus (HIV), herpes simplex virus (HSV) , rabies and Ebola virus etc.

- The main difference between bacteria and viruses is that bacteria can multiply by dividing themselves while a virus forces its host to produce thousands of copies of the virus.

- Antibiotics don't work against viruses. Researchers develop vaccines to fight them.

- The use of vaccines has led to a dramatic drop in illnesses and mortality associated with viral infections, such as mumps, rubella, polio, and measles.

- Melittin in bee venom has been found to act against viruses by rupturing their envelope.

- Our immune system is normally able to fight the bacteria and viruses invading our body

- Inflammation is a protective process of the body.

- Interestingly, beekeepers have increased levels of downregulating cytokines (IL10) compared to the general population.

- Bee venom is probably also an important part of the immune system of bees.

2. PREVENTIVE AND CURATIVE MEASURES

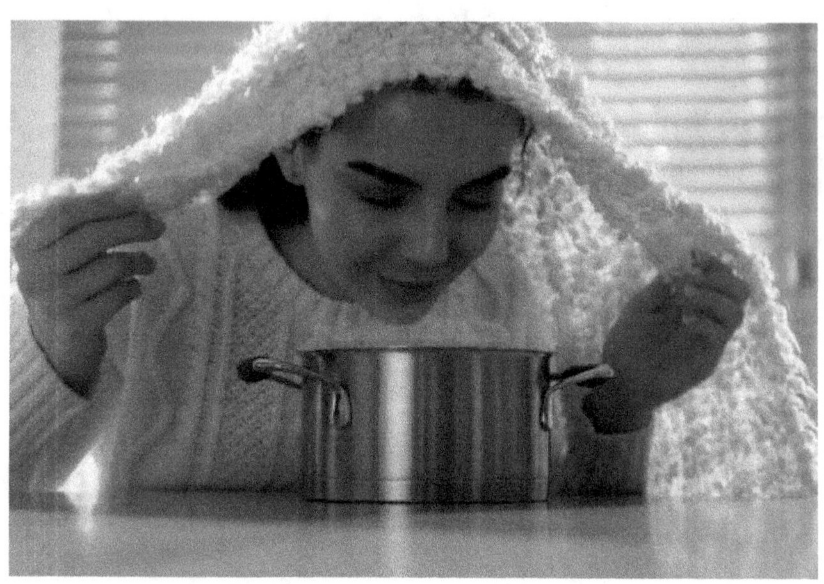

In this section you'll learn:

- When to take preventive and curative measures;

- What exactly to do;

- How to care for our digestive system;

- How to find the causes of our disorders;

When to take preventive and curative measures?

I don't feel the urge to take preventive measures all year long, only in the periods I know or I feel I'm susceptible to infectious diseases. I don't think either that is useful to be preventive all year long using honey as a "drug", propolis or bee venom.

It is time for preventive measures when one feels uncomfortable, depressed, has a headache, or a sore throat etc.

How can I tell that a pathogen is lurking or a longer lasting cold or some other infections are just around the corner?

Factors for preventive measures are:

I. Internal factors:
When I feel uncomfortable: I have a headache, sore throat, muscle tension, coated tongue, bad feeling or pain in my chest, stomach, guts; when I have diarrhea etc.

II. External factors:
1. End of winter/begin of spring – this is a generally acknowledged period for catching cold; the waiting rooms at the physicians' are full.

2. When travelling to different regions I'm often exposed to unknown viruses and bacteria, and after such travels my immune system may be weakened and I may fall ill.

3. In times when my close relations, colleagues get infected by something; everything seems okay if I stay healthy, but no doubt some pathogens have also tried to get a hold in me.

Preventive measures: hygiene, honey, propolis and bee venom

Depending on the gravity of the situation, I decide what extra hygiene measures to take and what bee products to use: honey, propolis or (rarely) bee stings.

I stop eating honey as usual, I eat it with curative goals in mind, which means I measure the daily amount of honey I ingest and after ingesting it I don't eat or drink anything else for half an hour so that the honey can have its beneficial effects. Consuming other food or drinks within half an hour could reduce or stop the production of hydrogen peroxide, which is one of the ways honey accomplishes its antimicrobial effects.

> *I make some diet changes, such as reducing carbohydrates, sugar and not drinking milk or eating milk products;*

I don't eat anything for 12-14 hours or even one or two days – except one or two tablespoons of honey at bedtime;

I take more care with my mouth hygiene: I gargle with baking soda, clean my coated tongue with a tablespoon, do nasal irrigation, brush my teeth several times a day.

I try to sleep more than usual.

Prevention for low or middle risk infection:

I assess a situation as being of low or middle risk when there are either light internal factors or external factors showing up. That means if I feel slightly bad or in my surroundings there are some people with infections. I try to figure out what may have caused the symptoms and I:

- do throat hygiene in the morning: gargling with baking soda: I put two teaspoons of Sodium bicarbonate in 250-300 ml (8,5-10 Fl. oz.) water and a pinch of salt and gargle with it at least twice a day or if the situation is worse, each half an hour); I do nasal irrigation (see in *How to do nasal irrigation?*, page 18) once a week; I clean my tongue with a tablespoon each morning when plaque can be seen on it and I brush my teeth whenever I feel the need for it during the day.

- select the right honey varietal for the given issue: either chestnut or acacia[i] for respiratory and digestive issues;

- take honey as a "drug", which means reducing its daily amount from 2-4 tablespoons to 2-4 teaspoons. I take the honey one hour before meals, so that it can work. In case of respiratory issues, **flu and cold**, I ingest honey with turmeric and black pepper, 2-3 half teaspoons a day. (See the exact use: Honey with turmeric and black pepper- **For digestive problems**: honey-chocolate in *Honey recipes*;)

- consider eating only some eggs at 10 a.m. and a small amount of resistant starch containing food (vegetables, unripe banana, cold fried potato, etc.) in the afternoon.

- drink herbal teas made with appropriate herbs (aniseed and fennel for stomach and intestine issues. A mixture of equal ratio of linden, elderflower and chamomile: for respiratory issues.);

- put lemon in my tea, but I don't put honey in it;

- do some exercises or/and walk in the fresh air for 10-20 minutes after meals;

- take in Vitamin B, C and D, zinc;

Curing Infections:

I consider myself to have an infection when two or more of the internal factors worsen (I feel really bad, depressed, I have a sore throat, muscle tension, I cough, have a runny nose, I have severe stomach or gut pain, bloating, flatulence, diarrhea etc.)

---

[i] You may have other local honey varietals available for the given issues.

In such situations, I do what I described for the prevention of low and middle risk infections including hygiene measures (in case of flu and cold, if I can, I do nasal irrigation several times and inhalation with herbs, honey – See the *interview with Dr. Stangaciu*, page 41), plus:

- If I have fever I don't reduce it until it's within normal ranges 38,5-41,6 C;

- *In case of **digestive infections** (when I have bloating, flatulence, diarrhea) I take a teaspoon of propolis tincture (40-50 drops) in about 20-30 ml water three times a day (in the morning, at noon and in the evening) half an hour before meals; In case of **flu or cold** I only take the half of the dose and only once a day: half teaspoon (20-25 drops) of propolis in the morning in 20-30 ml of water);*

- I do 24 hour fasting for 2 consecutive days: I eat once a day at 10.am. some eggs or food that helps move the bile into the small intestine;

- I skip honey during the day; I only take one or two teaspoons at bedtime (chestnut/linden/acacia);

- I consume some good quality liquid (not powder) probiotics from the pharmacy;

- I let my wife do bee venom massage on my spinal meridians and let her sting me with bees at the points where issues can be detected. (See details in the *Bee Venom* section, page 129)

- If my situation doesn't change in 3 days, I reassess the situation and decide whether to use larger amounts of propolis: 50 drops in 20-30 ml of water at once; or to use some royal jelly (if I have some) 3x1 gram. I raise the number of bee stings on the problematic points of my spinal meridians.

- And of course recovering from any infection includes drinking plenty of water, lemonade and herbal teas, resting, getting plenty of sleep, staying warm.

I rarely exceed 2-4 days with these measures.

The above system works very well for me and may work for you too. But it is also possible that you may need to develop, or you already have, different preventive measures.

If an infection appears again and again it is important to think about lifestyle changes and visit a physician (See in chapter <u>Making Lifestyle changes</u>, page 168).

Take care of your digestive system

The right diet and good digestion play the most important part in our health. Being aware of digestive issues and taking care of the digestive system is as important as hygienic measures.

Following the latest research on nutrients can pay out, especially if you have constant inflammation in your body (high levels of inflammation markers).

Reducing the daily intake of carbohydrates, even honey (1-2 tablespoons - 30-80 grams a day) and fruits can be an important measure.

If you have reflux, constant bloating, flatulence, irritable bowel syndrome, etc, change your diet.

In many cases, a low carb diet and ketogenic diet helps to reduce high levels of inflammation markers or high levels of cholesterol.

I won't give details about diets in this book, I can only say that one of the turning points in my health happened when I changed to a low carb diet.

Helping lazy digestion

I thought that having a stool once in 2 or 3 days was normal. You can read here and there that this may be very individual, but when I asked a specialist whether it's normal having such slow digestion, he was quite alarmed and told me that 2-3 times, but at least once a day, one should have a stool.

He gave me the advice to eat more fibre and drink lukewarm water. But all this only mildly improved the issue.

Then I did some experiments: eating some food containing resistant starch and trying a hydrotherapeutic technique – putting a towel soaked with cold water on my belly to contract the dilated intestines helped me with lazy digestion.

Helping your microbiome with resistant starch

Resistant starch can be digested only in the large intestine, which means it is perfect food for the microbiome just like the oligosaccharide part of honey.

It helps feed the good bacteria in our gut and increases the production of a short-chain fatty acid called butyrate which has anti-inflammatory and anti-cancer properties, too. It can help with weight loss and benefit heart health.

As resistant starch is not transformed and absorbed in our small intestines, it does not increase insulin levels.

Eating resistant starch on a daily basis seems to help my digestion.

It may seem strange, but research demonstrates that resistant starch comes about[7] in the wholly cooked then cooled pasta, rice, potatoes, it is present in raw potatoes, raw oats, unripe bananas, in deep frozen and toasted bread, in beans, peas.

Keep also in mind that even if they contain resistant starch, most of the carbohydrates in these foods aren't resistant and will be transformed and absorbed in your small intestines.

Raw potato starch though it is processed food can serve as a good source of resistant starch (80%).

Put one or two teaspoons of potato starch powder in yogurt or water.

A "tasty" recipe for a kind of instant soup:

100 ml of water (room temperature), 2- teaspoons of raw potato starch powder, one pinch of salt, a pinch of fresh black pepper, a pinch of vitamin-c.

Even in periods when I follow a low carb diet, I eat some food containing resistant starch.

A hydrotherapeutic practice

A towel soaked with cold tap water wrung out then placed on the lower part of the belly from side to side can help with contracting the large intestines if they are dilated and therefore lazy.

In my case, it helped already on the first day I applied the towel for about 10-15 minutes.

It might have also activated my appendix, an organ considered for long time by science as useless.

Latest research suggests that the appendix may play an important role in reestablishing our original microbiome, as it is a reservoir of our gut bacteria.[8]

Cold showers also have a constraining effect on the large intestines when letting the water pour on your belly from side to side.

Diarrhea

Diarrhea may be a sign that some pathogens, like microbes, fungi, worms, or undesired chemicals, antibiotics, or indigestible small objects have entered the digestive system and the intestines want to get rid of them. If the diarrhea lasts only for a short time (1-2) days it can be seen as a healthy cleansing process.

Help this process by fasting (if not contraindicated for you – see *Fasting* below) and taking propolis tincture, 30-40 drops in about 20-

30 ml water three times a day (in the morning, at noon and in the evening, if not fasting, half an hour before meals.)

Drink plenty of water. You may also take supplements of important minerals and vitamins to deal with their loss caused by the diarrhea.

Regular fasting and the use of propolis in such a way may help even if the diarrhea is caused by Irritable Bowel Syndrome. In such cases, when not fasting a low FODMAP-diet (fermentable oligo- di- mono-saccharides and polyols) is also advised.

You may experience diarrhea from milk products or meals produced in countries where they use antibiotics in animal farming. Try to avoid such food if you have concluded that your diarrhea may be caused by such.

If the diarrhea is recurring or lasts more than a few days it can damage your health or even be lethal. In any case of long lasting or recurring diarrhea drink plenty of water and visit a doctor!

Fasting

Fasting helps important bodily functions. It reduces insulin levels, and initiates cellular repair processes like autophagy.

Fasting can be very helpful when ill, infected or just for prevention.

During fasting the levels of growth hormone skyrocket, increasing as much as 5-fold. Besides all these, possibly the most important is that there are changes in the function of genes related to longevity and protection against disease.[9]

When fasting, it is important to consider your preconditions. In my case, years ago I concluded that my gallbladder stones were caused by a poor diet, and after changing my diet to help the bile move from the gallbladder into the intestines before noon (!) my gallbladder stones soon stopped being an issue. (See details in chapter *A "half success"* story) That's why when doing intermittent fasting (eating only once/24 hours 2 times a week) it is important for me to eat that one meal before noon in the morning or at 10 a.m.

Women should be more cautious than men when fasting as fasting may have an impact on their hormone balance and it can affect menstruation, elevated insulin levels, etc.

Fasting is also a bad idea if you're pregnant or breastfeeding.

Underweight people or people with a history of eating disorders should consult a physician before fasting.

Intermittent Fasting

Fasting can be challenging and for most people it is hard to stick to it. But intermittent fasting seems to be a more psychologically and physically viable way. You can choose and experiment with different forms of IF.

Intermittent fasting means splitting the day or week into eating and fasting periods.

During the fasting periods, you eat either very little or nothing at all.

The most popular methods of IF:

The 16/8 method: it involves restricting your daily eating period to 8 hours, such as 10 a.m.- 6 p.m. Then you fast for 16 hours in between. (You can also try other variations: 12/12, 18/6, 20/4)

Eat-Stop-Eat: This involves fasting for 24 hours, once or twice a week, for example by not eating from breakfast (10 a.m.) one day until breakfast (10 a.m.) the next day.

The 5:2 diet: you consume only 450–600 calories on two nonconsecutive days of the week. But you eat normally the other 5 days.

As long as you don't compensate by eating much more during the eating periods, all of these methods should cause weight loss or trigger the functions mentioned earlier.

The 16/8 method is the simplest and easiest to stick to. But when you are infected or feel ill consider the Eat-Stop-Eat method for 1-2 days.

How to find out the causes of our disorders

When we feel ill, have headaches, a runny nose, flatulence, stomach-aches or any pain, it is good to counteract it with a cure, change of diet, fasting. But it is equally important to search for the causes.

Usually when we fall ill we don't think too much about the reasons. We are concerned and focused on the issue itself. And it isn't easy to determine the causes if our day is overloaded with many different actions, tasks, foods, drinks, meetings, briefings etc.

> *Searching for the reasons is helpful, even if we don't discover the exact cause of a certain pain, nausea etc. It'll make us more conscious of our daily routines and in many cases, we will figure out the causes.*

Let me explain this through a personal story:

My wife's 'heart issue'

One morning my wife was complaining of accelerated heartbeats and arrhythmia, which was astonishing as she lives a healthy life, eating mostly quality food and exercising or jogging regularly. She told me that she'd been experiencing these symptoms for a week. We both got a bit scared and I told her that she should visit a cardiologist as soon as possible.

But she was to travel to a conference that same day and was gone for a few days. The next morning, being home alone, I found that there was no ground coffee at home for my morning drink. I only found some instant coffee. I don't really like instant coffe, but as a cup of morning coffee with acacia honey is important for me, I prepared one cup of it. A bit time later, I felt my heart start to accelerate and it seemed as if it was leaving out some beats, too. The whole thing was very strange and annoying, something I had never experienced before. It did not last too long, maybe 1-2 minutes, so I forgot about it by evening when I talked to my wife on the phone. The next morning, the same thing happened. This time I tried to think about what might have caused the unusual and frightening symptoms.

In the evening, when talking to my wife on the phone, I asked her whether she still had the heart issue she had been telling me about two days earlier. She told me she hadn't had any symptoms since she had left.

Then I asked her whether she'd been drinking instant coffee the previous week when she was at home. The answer was yes, as she had been hurrying in the mornings.

The next morning I didn't prepare coffee from the instant coffee, but drank a herbal tea with my daily morning honey. And I had no heart issues!

After buying our usual brand of coffee, I threw out the one which had probably caused the heart acceleration and arrhythmia. And neither my wife nor I have experienced that again.

This is a good example of how easily we can consume (or do) things that are harmful to us, without even being aware of what might have caused the problem. When we carry on with harmful habits for weeks, months or even years, the inevitable will come.

Determining the causes of our disorders

In many cases we ignore signs, as they aren't too shocking and we can live with them. But ignoring them is a weakness which will only allow the invaders to gain a stronger foothold.

Becoming aware of our body's signs is key. The next time you realize that something is strange or different, don't put off asking some questions.

Questions help

If we feel pain, our body lets us know that something harmful is happening inside. It's sensible to listen to these signs and not to ignore them.

First of all, describe to yourself in a few words or phrases what you realize when experiencing pain or other signs of illness.

This kind of objective description can be applied to the consistency of your stool, urine etc. as well, when they appear to be different from usual.

For example: "I feel a slight pain in my belly on the right. It spreads further downwards. I have felt this pain before (or I have never felt this pain before), when I ate some…… When putting my hands on my belly it feels like it's being inflated. My belly is hard. etc.

It's important that you don't mix your emotions or prejudices into this description. Be objective and focus on the "topic", which means don't let your thoughts get distracted from the subject, i.e. the above thoughts, when distracted, could be: "I fear that I have a peptic ulcer and I'm scared because my father died from peptic ulcers. I loved my father. He was caring and we played a lot in our garden. I remember once…."

Then answering the following questions may help us to discover the causes of certain pains, nausea, headaches, etc. The more detailed the answers, the more likely you'll find out the reasons and causes. But don't worry if you can't figure it out exactly. Going through the process of asking questions and answering them can make us more conscious of our daily routines and life. You may write down your answers, but it's not necessary.

Of course, you don't need to go through all these questions, but look through the most obvious ones concerning your issue.

What may cause the............ (whatever inconvenience you feel, you may fill in the gap: headache, stomach pain etc.)?

What did I eat/drink today/yesterday/in the previous days? You can describe in detail your servings, or even the circumstances.

Where have I been? How did I get there? (by car, public transport, on foot etc.)

With whom did I meet?

What did I do today or in the previous days?

What exercises did I do?

Was there anything strange in my day or in the days before?

Have I slept well?

Summary:

- In periods for preventive measures make some diet changes,

- Stop eating honey as usual, eat it with curative goals in mind.

- Take more care with your mouth hygiene: gargle with baking soda, clean the coated tongue with a tablespoon, do nasal irrigation, sleep more;

- Take care of your digestive system by reducing carbohydrates (sugar, starch) and by helping your microbiome;

- A low carb diet and ketogenic diet helps to reduce high levels of inflammation markers;

- Resistant starch can be digested only in the large intestine, which means it is perfect food for the microbiome;

- If your digestion is lazy, hydrotherapeutic practices may help (towel soaked with cold water, cold showers on your belly);

- Fasting helps important bodily functions. It reduces insulin levels, and initiates cellular repair processes like autophagy;

- Becoming aware of our body's signs is key; Answering some questions may help us to discover the causes of certain pains, nausea, headaches.

3. ARE BEEKEEPERS PROTECTED FROM PATHOGENS?

AN INTERVIEW

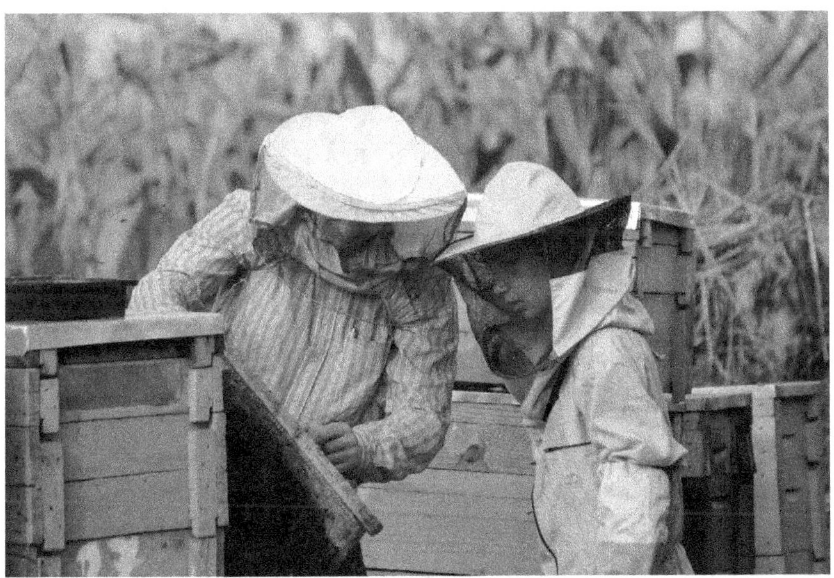

This interview made for beekeeping journals[10] summarizes and provides an idea about our immune system, bee products and apitherapy techniques. It's worth reading it to understand the message of Dr. Stangaciu message, a renowned apitherapist and author of books and articles on that subject.[i]

[i] **General Secretary of the** International Federation of Apitherapy, **Honorary President of the** German Apitherapy Society, **President of the** Romanian Apitherapy Society; **His courses and activity see: apitherapy.com**

Dr. Stangaciu can you tell us about our immune system? How does it work?

First of all when talking about the immune system, most people think of the white blood cells, the leukocytes, which is correct, but in fact, our body has many protective layers. We have energetic layers, like our planet has a magnetic field. We have similar things, like meridians or our aura, which is the first layer of physical protection.

Then we have another protective layer: the skin. It provides mechanical protection, but there is also biochemical protection on top, in and under the skin, the layers of fats.

Immediately under the skin and mucosa (internal "skins"), like nose, mouth, digestive, respiratory, and vaginal mucosa, there is a whole layer of macrophages and neutrophils which also belong to the immune system. They are specialized to protect us from invasion by viruses, bacteria, fungi, and parasites. The same kind of protection is around our intestines, especially around our large intestine. These are special areas with concentrated lymphocytes. 70% of our body's lymphocytes are around our intestines!

But we are protected even at a cellular level, aren't we?

Yes, every single cell of our body has, more or less, the power to defend itself. If they are healthy, cells can produce interferon, a kind of protein which can block viruses or bacteria. When a virus enters the cell and multiplies, it creates a lot of free radicals, which help viruses by breaking the cell, just as if they were small scissors, microscopically speaking. If the cell is full of antioxidants, these free radicals are quickly blocked and the virus cannot multiply or cannot do so much damage.

All I want to say is it's very important to help each of the many levels of our protection and not just one of them. The outermost level is psycho-emotional protection: being depressed, fearful, worried, jealous, angry and so on affect our nervous system. Then the nervous system affects the endocrine system, it overworks the hypophysis and other endocrine glands, like the adrenal glands, and then adrenalin and cortisol are not produced correctly, and the immune system is weakened.

Scientifically it's already known and confirmed in large studies of psycho-neuro-immunology that these problems affect our immune system. Unfortunately, in this time of social isolation and other measures adopted by our governments, which have their own logic, excessive isolation will make people depressed, angry and fearful, diminishing their immune system. And immune system health is most important to fight any kind of virus.

The virus itself is not problem. Let's say, it is 10% of the problem, 90% of the issue is the immune system. Statistics from all over the world show that about 95% of people infected with SARS-COV 2 experience no problems. They may be carrying the virus, but they don't have any symptoms or only mild ones. Moreover, from the 5% who get ill only about 2% have severe issues. The big question is, if we want to think with a clear mind, "Why do only these 2% have problems?" We have some answers: i.e they have too many comorbidities (diabetes, heart issues, capillary fragility, obesity, etc.). But they also have a weakened immune system. This is the main cause of Covid-19!

And vice versa, we can ask the question: "Why don't 95% percent of the infected people get severely ill?" And if we have the answers, we can develop solutions for helping the other 5% who get ill.

Could you talk a bit about which tissues and organs are part of our immune system?

We have Peyer's patches in our intestines. Lymphatic nodes are present all over the body. Then the red bone marrow is particularly important, especially in the long bones where the white blood cells, red blood cells and the platelets are produced. Then we have the thymus. And we have special lymphoid organs around the nose or in the throat like tonsils and so on. We have also the spleen. All these organs are places where the immune system trains, develops and multiplies…. If they function well they also cooperate. Let's say the virus just arrived in the nose, then the white blood cells must be able to go very quickly from all over the body to this area, to the nose. For this we must improve the fluidity of the blood and the lymph, making it possible for the white blood cells to travel very quickly to the affected area, in this case, into the tissues of the nose.

How can we improve the fluidity of blood and lymph?

One way is to change your diet, avoiding food that reduces blood and lymph fluidity. Another very good method is to increase the body's temperature or to help the fever. In a nutshell, that is the immune system. I advise everyone to do her or his own research or read about the immune system and everyone can find out what makes your immune system happy in order to work properly.

What about beekeepers, are they protected against COVID 19 to a certain extent?

Well, as far as we know, they have no problems with COVID 19. We know about very few beekeepers infected with the coronavirus or else they got rid of it very quickly. In China, they did a survey of 5119 beekeepers and about 112 patients receiving apitherapy and none of them died. This is the first study on this topic conducted in China confirming the immunity of beekeepers. Of course, we need further studies to come to a definite conclusion.

Why are beekeepers so well protected?

Well, beekeepers use bee products like pollen, bee bread, melittin (from bee stings), and honey, which have polyphenols and organic acids, or they breathe in volatile substances from the beehive air, beeswax or propolis. Then the royal jelly and the drone larvae (Apilarnil) contain a lot of useful regenerative substances. Royal jelly has telomerase, as do pollen and beebread, too. So all these active substances are good nutrients and they protect us against viruses as well.

Let's talk about how we can improve our immune system with bee products and lifestyle changes.

We have to consider that our immune system can be affected by many factors. A good therapist first needs to identify all these factors, and then need to deal with them one by one. The patient will thus heal much faster.

Stress is an especially important factor and these days when all the TV channels and media are full of stressful information about Covid-19, people are scared. This raises cortisol levels in the blood and downregulates the immune system.

Free radicals also impair immune system function. They can be found in fried food, fast food, they can come from smoking or from the polluted air of big cities.

If **the blood and lymph are "sticky** or **muddy"** then the "soldiers" of our immune system (the white blood cells) cannot "travel" fast enough, just as mentioned in the first part of this interview. Imagine an army with well-trained soldiers, but they are in a muddy, icy, snowy forest where they cannot move properly to approach and fight the enemy.

Dehydration is a major issue for the immune system. Even if you feel that you drink enough water you may be dehydrated, for different reasons i.e. eating too much protein that requires lots of water to be digested, or you may lose water through your lungs when doing physical exercise, etc.

How can I check whether I am dehydrated?

There are some physical signs. If you have constipation this may be a sign of dehydration.

It is good to look at your tongue and if you can see the traces of the teeth around on the margin, or if you pinch your skin on your arm and if it doesn't go back quickly but stays a bit pinched for some moments, it means you need to drink more water.

If your urine is very light-yellow and doesn't smell bad, that usually means that you are well hydrated.

If we find that we are dehydrated, how can we drink more water without it being expelled from our body quickly?

You can add a very small amount of lemon juice and honey to the water and the body will absorb it more easily. Or you can take a small pinch of salt when drinking water.

It's not about drinking large amounts of water, but about having enough water in your body so that blood flows well and your immune system can work properly: the leucocytes must be able to rapidly get to the places where the intruders have to be eliminated.

Lack of oxygen: that can be corrected with different methods, one is regular and proper, tonifying movements in fresh air, walking, jogging, trekking, swimming, etc.

Poor diet is another problem. If people don't eat enough vitamins (B, C, D, etc.), enzymes, minerals, proteins, fats or if they just make poor food choices (too many carbohydrates, sugar, HFCs, or they get too little protein, fat, etc.) it is also a problem for our health. But there is no rule that everybody should eat only fruits, or vegetables or only proteins or fats. Chinese Medicine or Ayurveda give particularly good advice in this respect, which are personally tailored.

Fatigue: The immune system needs lots of energy, so you need rest and good sleep, at least 7-8 hours a day.

Microorganisms also affect our immune system; we live together with many of them, which help us in our functioning. But we may be attacked by many co-infections, parasites, fungi, viruses, or bacteria and if so, the immune system cannot cope with all of them, it will fail to protect us.

Hygiene (e.g. washing your hands properly) is very important, but internal hygiene is even more important. It can be only accomplished if our kidneys work well and they eliminate the water-soluble toxins. Likewise, the intestines and liver must work well, too, as they eliminate the fat- soluble toxins. If the lungs work properly, they will eliminate many volatile toxins . But the skin is also eliminating toxins through the sweat and sebaceous glands.

Capillary fragility: In my opinion this is one of the greatest problems in Covid 19, because when you read about the deaths, most patients had micro-thrombosis. First, they experience micro-bleeding, which triggers the creation of blood clots in the small blood vessels, like in a heart attack or a stroke.

How can beehive products help us?

We can facilitate the elimination of toxins i.e. by drinking lemon juice (one- two lemons/day) in 500 ml of (40-42 °C, 104-107°F) water with 2-3 teaspoons of honey. We call this mixture lemonade – well known to each of us – and it has enough water to clear the water-soluble toxins and enough citric acid, which together with the honey's soft organic acids, will help the cleansing of fat-soluble toxins from our body. And this is an especially important point. We cannot eliminate fat-soluble toxins with only water. Honey and all other foods that contain organic acids can help, like this quite easy-to-make lemonade.

Honey, containing enzymes and energy, can help with many things, including with a good rest as well. If you take one spoonful of honey at bedtime, it will help with sleep.

The sugars in honey consist of small molecules already broken down by the bees. Potatoes for example consist of large starch molecules, which first need to be broken down by our body; in honey the bees have already done this. This is one of the enormous advantages of honey, especially for very tired or very ill people who do not have enough enzymes and/or energy to break down the long chain carbohydrates.

What about pollen? I usually have diarrhea from eating pollen, what may be the cause and how can I avoid it?

Pollen can help supplement minerals, varied proteins, and vitamins, various *Lactobacillus* species, telomerase etc., but if not stored correctly as beebread or deep frozen, it may develop fungi, which can cause diarrhea. To avoid this problem, one of the best methods to store the raw pollen is in the freezer, at minus 16 degrees Celsius, immediately after its collection.

Just take out only the amount you need from the freezer, then put the rest right back.

Dried pollen is not so good as many volatile parts and many antioxidants have been eliminated from it.

We believed for a long time that beebread is made by the bees to make the pollen digestible, but it's made just for a proper storage, isn't it?

The exina of the pollen which serves as a protection for the pollen it is not broken down in bee bread either.

Yes, that's a relatively new observation of an American researcher named Kirk Douglas. If you look under the microscope, the exina of the pollen, be it raw pollen or beebread, is not broken down. It is a hard protection that cannot be destroyed by our stomach acids or other enzymes of our body. It is suggested that it will be broken down only in the large intestine. There may be certain bacteria capable of breaking through the exina.

My hypothesis is that there are certain bacteria gathered by the bees from the environment (from stagnant, muddy water or compost) which help them with the digestion of the pollen.

Sure, bees eventually can digest pollen and use it in their body. In fact, this is exceptionally good news, as its nutrients and active substances (including telomerase) arrive in the large intestine – thus helping the regeneration of our own telomeres (which can be found at the ends of our chromosomes).

You are advocating the use of large amounts of royal jelly…

…Royal Jelly is antiviral, antifungal, and antibacterial. It helps the immune system, it helps the body to produce red and white blood cells and platelets. It can heal severe illnesses. I know people in the recent pandemic in Germany who recovered from Covid 19 by taking large amounts of Royal Jelly – 50-60 ml/day, administered 2-5 ml hourly during the day.

Let us have a look, what if someone has got symptoms of some infections, what can he or she do?

Well, some symptoms at the beginning of an infection let's say in case of Covid 19, may be running nose, coughing, vomiting, diarrhea or fever, all of these are normal functions of the body which tries to eliminate the viruses or other pathogens.

We can use mechanical ways to help our body in the elimination of the virus.

Heat destroys most pathogens; viruses for example are destroyed at 56 degrees Celsius in 10-15 minutes, which is amazingly fast. That is because viruses, like other pathogens are made of proteins, and proteins, when heated, coagulate, get denatured, change their structure and thus become inactive. Even if the virus arrives in the nose, in the mouth, in the throat, in the lungs or in the bronchi, in the first one-two days it does not normally come in contact with the body cells, because they "land" first in the mucus that covers the whole respiratory and digestive systems. After contact with the virus, a healthy respiratory system will start to produce even more mucus, a thin, "runny", "watery" mucus, which can be eliminated more easily from the nose, sinuses or lungs through expectoration than a thick mucus.

A wet sauna is a particularly good idea in prevention or at the first phase of an infection (runny nose, sore throat, etc.) because it combines heat and humidity.

The old way that was used by our grandparents, the traditional inhalation is also exceptionally good. You need just a towel, hot water, propolis tincture and honey to inhale "medicinal" vapors that will help your body a lot.

Besides these physical methods, chemical methods, such as those suggested by our governments are also useful: the use of detergents, soaps etc. which is good for our hygiene. Of course, you cannot ingest detergents. You can though use soft organic acids, which are present in the beehive products too, because they also damage pathogens through direct contact (the acids "burn" at the molecular level). You can gargle with honey diluted in some saline solution, or put it in hot water when inhaling it.

When inhaling honey, won't the enzymes in it be destroyed?
They will be destroyed but, in this case, we need the acids from honey which are not destroyed by heat.

But you can use a nebulizer, too, which is a device used by people with asthma and which doesn't use heat but it produces fog from the solution put in it, at room temperature.

You can use the following recipe by Dr. Doina Cojocaru from Romania:

3 ml of physiological serum (saline water solution)

0,5 ml honey (honeydew honey or other antibacterial honey – chestnut, linden, eucalyptus etc.)

10 drops of propolis tincture (20-30%)

In the case of a bacterial infection, add max. 1 drop of volatile oil (thyme, fir, eucalyptus…).

What if the illness worsens, can we also use bee products?

Well, propolis has an anti-oedema effect and in the case of lung diseases, when too much water fills them it may help a lot.

It may also happen that people get hypoxia – low levels of oxygen – because of low levels of hemoglobin (in red blood cells) or because the virus may have destroyed the red blood cells as well. For these issues, we can increase the production of red blood cells by using royal jelly, bee bread and fresh frozen bee pollen. These bee products contain substances which stimulate the stem cells in the red bone marrow to produce more blood cells.

Scientific studies clearly show that both royal jelly and propolis help with the use of oxygen in the cells, especially if the patient is getting enough rest, sleeping more and reducing stress levels, thus overall consuming less oxygen.

Well I think only one interview doesn't allow us to cover everything about beehive products. I hope we have raised the readers' interest in very effective and interesting methods and useful remedies. I'd like to thank you Dr. Stangaciu for this exceptional interview!

Thank you and I wish with all my heart for you and the readers to stay healthy!

Summary

- Our immune system provides complex protection, even at the cellular level;

- It is important to help each level of our immune system, including the psycho-emotional level by reducing stress, fear etc;

- We can improve the fluidity of our blood and lymph by avoiding dehydration and drinking enough water;

- The immune system needs lots of energy, so you need rest and good sleep, at least 7-8 hours a day;

- We can facilitate the elimination of toxins i.e. by drinking lemon juice;

- Pollen can help supplement minerals, varied proteins, and vitamins, various *Lactobacillus* species;

- Royal Jelly is antiviral, antifungal, and antibacterial. It helps the body to produce red and white blood cells and platelets;

- Heat destroys most pathogens; viruses for example are destroyed at 56 degrees Celsius in 10-15 minutes;

- A wet sauna, inhalation, and a nebulizer are each a good idea for prevention or at the first phase of an infection (runny nose, sore throat, etc.);

- Both royal jelly and propolis help with the use of oxygen in the cells;

BEE PRODUCTS

4. HONEY

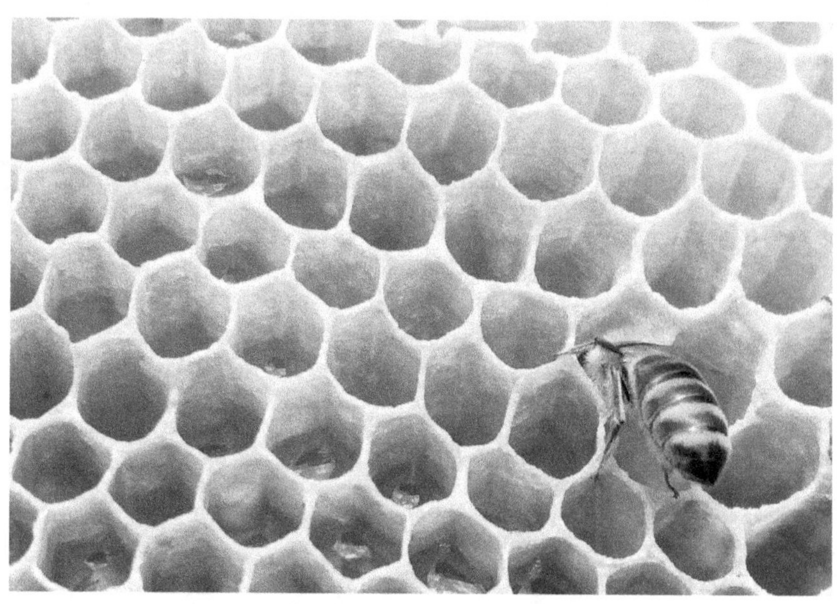

In this section you'll learn:

- Where honey comes from;
- How to use honey;
- Whether honey is superior to table sugar;
- How much honey to eat;
- How to teach our brain to give up sugar-rich food;
- Whether honey is for diabetics;

My praise of honey

When one experiences the benefits of consuming honey (that is pure, ripe, raw and not adulterated honey!) she or he will admire it as a super food, working exceptionally for our health, regulating our immune system and giving prompt energy to our brain and body without damaging it – if consumed moderately!

When reading about all the benefits of honey it might be tempting to throw caution to the winds and consume vast quantities of it, which wouldn't be a good idea.

I have to warn you to be cautious and not overeat honey just as I do sometimes when I cannot resist the "seduction" especially when extracting fresh, delicious, aroma-rich honey from the combs.

If we eat more honey than our liver can store as glycogen (about 1-2.5 tablespoons of honey at once), the rest stays in our blood, raising insulin and sugar levels.

But interestingly, a small amount of honey does not increase blood sugar levels as much as the same dose of table sugar (sucrose) or HFCS – no large insulin spike is triggered by honey in our blood.[11]

Where honey comes from

Flowers produce nectar, while aphids secrete honeydew as they feed on plant sap. The bees collect both nectar and honeydew as they are rich in sugar.

Both nectar and honeydew contain 30-90% water. That would spoil over time and that's why bees turn them into honey.

When nectar is brought into the hive, worker bees start ventilating with their wings and move the nectar drops by regurgitating them from one hexagonal cell to other. They dry out the nectar and during the process they enrich it with enzymes from their glands, which cleave complex sugars into simple ones. They add other substances, like the antibacterial peptide, defensin-1; glucose oxidase (GOX) – the enzyme responsible for the formation of hydrogen peroxide (H2O2), which plays a major role in the antiviral and antibacterial properties of honey; and major royal jelly proteins (MRJP), like albumin.

> *All in all you'll find 181 substances in honey! And this is what distinguishes honey from other "sweeteners". These substances may help the sugars in honey being metabolized differently from table sugar or HFCS.*

The honey is ready when most of the water has been dried out of the nectar or honeydew and less than 18-19% remains. Then they seal it with wax.

Appreciating honey

Many years ago I appreciated honey only a bit more than table sugar. Just as generally people do. All in all, besides its sweetness, it has more aroma than sugar. I thought of this just as others do, even though I've been keeping bees and regularly eating honey since my childhood.

But two essential experiences made me think of honey in a different way. The first one was when honey helped me with my stomach issues you can read below and the second one is in the chapter *Honey for insomnia*, page 96).

But honey can be appreciated for its beneficial effects in wound healing as well: one of my beekeeper colleagues suffered a grave accident with his motorcycle. His doctor told him his injury would take a long time to heal. The physician was quite astonished when the beekeeper showed up with his injuries healed much earlier than expected. He used honey on his injuries!

A "half" success story: Canola honey reduces reflux and inhibits bacteria in our stomach:

I tried out many things to sooth my reflux and reduce my stomach pain about 15 years ago. The phenomenon of reflux came into my life when, as a vegetarian I would eat food without watching its carbohydrate, starch and added sugar content. I ate lots of wheat, rice, potatoes, milk and food with added sugar. I know now that this was a problem.

I could only eat a teaspoon or less of honey a day without having almost unbearable stomach issues (pain or reflux).

I tried many alkalizing foods, plants, powders etc. that worked well for a while. But as the basic causes, which were – as it turned out later – a peptic ulcer and gallbladder stones, were probably aggravated, the pain just wouldn't disappear by eating "alkalizing" food.

I was somewhat skeptical when a beekeeper colleague told me that one of his customers, who had reflux bought 10 kilos of canola honey at a time because it reduced his reflux and soothed his stomach pain. I had a hard time believing this, because canola honey, while less acidic (with a pH of about 4.0) than other honey varietals, is still acidic. At that time I didn't have much experience with canola honey as in my region we had just a little and we didn't harvest it.

But I gave it a try. I got some canola honey from my colleague and ingested a teaspoon of it. And I really didn't feel any pain in my stomach, moreover it felt kind of soothing. Then I tried a tablespoon of canola honey and my stomach felt fine. This was almost unbelievable after a whole year of reflux and stomach issues. The relief brought by canola honey was a real discovery for me.

But things got a bit more complicated.

I have to add that I hadn't yet made essential changes in my diet at that time, however I tried to "alkalize" myself which was then a trend.

My reflux and stomach pain didn't disappear completely though I regained some hope and self-confidence that it could be healed in a natural way.

But there was a problem with the decreased stomach pain and "self-confidence": it made me procrastinate searching for the real causes of the illness and I went on consuming soft drinks, carbohydrate- and starch-rich food.

Night after night I woke up terrible spasm-like pains in my stomach and on right part of my upper abdomen which would last for 2-3 hours.

Then things got even worse. While driving home after a really delicious and spicy meal in an Indian restaurant, I felt such a terrible pain in my chest, probably from reflux, that I thought it was a heart attack. I soon drove to the hospital where they diagnosed gallbladder stones.

I was advised not to eat fats, cabbage, spicy food etc. and that as soon as possible to visit a surgeon to remove my gallbladder, as the only efficient way to get rid of the stones is an operation.

Of course I didn't want to get rid from one of my organs, so first I tried a gallbladder cleansing technique with olive oil. I had to ingest half a liter of olive oil with lemon juice and honey. The first bits were delicious, but ingesting half a liter of it was a terrible experience. Then the next morning I had thorough diarrhea. Such a cleansing helped me for a week or two and I was spasm-free at night, but my reflux was still present. When checked by my physician neither the stones nor the basic pain had disappeared after 2 months of carrying out this olive oil cleanse several times.

My stomach pain first disappeared for a "longer" time (2-3 weeks) from a propolis cure that I describe in the *Propolis* section, page 115). But without overall diet change, the discomfort came back even after the propolis cure.

This is a good example that illnesses are complex issues. You cannot be successful only by changing "something" in your routine. You have to make substantial changes to achieve long-lasting effects. A remedy or drug will only hide the symptoms if the basic causes or habits aren't cleared up and changed. And that's the trick!

If I had accepted the general advice ones gets for treating reflux or "taking care" with her or his gallbladder stones, which is to ingest pills against reflux or have her or his gallbladder removed (in many cases it is advisable to have the gallbladder removed as "stones" in it can cause tumors as well!), the symptoms probably would have disappeared, but my peptic ulcer might have remained.

Of course a good doctor could help by advising some diet and lifestyle changes. Unfortunately, that rarely happens, or if you get some diet advice at the doctor's it is mostly general and not personally tailored to you. It's probably not a realistic expectation from our health care system to consider our uniqueness, as physicians and clinics are overloaded.

My bilious attacks disappeared in a few weeks after making substantial changes in my diet. But my peptic ulcer stayed with me for a few more months, until I made a propolis and canola honey cure.

At my last check-up I still had some gallbladder-stones, but they were apparently smaller and fewer. I hope they will eventually disappear completely.

Where to buy honey and how to check whether honey has been adulterated or not?

As honey can be adulterated, overheated and overfiltered, or it may contain remnants from chemicals used against pests – the honey label doesn't tell us much about it – it is crucial to buy honey from a reliable source.

Even if the honey is labelled as organic or raw honey, it may have been overheated when packaged.

The descriptions on the internet for checking for whether honey is real don't work, as the techniques of adulteration are very developed. There are huge factories in Asian countries producing 'honey'.

Neither will a simply lab test help. That's why isn't easy to check the honey coming across borders. For a reliable test you'd need Nuclear Magnetic Resonance (NMR) profiling. This technique compares the spectral features of authentic honey with the sample in question.

> *The best is to use local honey purchased from a local bee-keeper that you trust, at the market or from your neighborhood.*

But there is a simple test you can make when buying liquid honey: put a sample of it in the fridge for several weeks. If it crystallizes over the time it's pure honey, if not, it is made of sugar syrup. Unfortunately not every form of adulteration can be checked with this method!

Which honey is best?

I advocate the use of local honey varietals which I think is the best choice for healing purposes. It hasn't undergone long transportation, it's less probable that it is pasteurized, etc.

Your local honey varietals may differ from mine. To find out what is available in your area go to the local market or visit a beekeeper. Some will be happy to show you around their apiary and talk about honey varietals or their craft.

It is generally believed that darker honeys contain more healing power then lighter ones, because they possess higher concentrations of antioxidants, minerals, enzymes etc. But, that's not a rule of thumb.

Once you have found out what types of honey are characteristic for your region, you may find out about their healing powers as well.

The consistency, sugariness and healing properties of honey depend largely on its flower sources.

> *Honey is primarily classified by the type of plant the nectar or honeydew was collected from.*

For instance "Lime (Linden) honey" or "acacia honey", means the nectar comes from the flower of the plant with the same name. In the case of "pine honey' it was made of the honeydew collected on pine trees.

Honey from just one nectar source is "unifloral" honey – like canola or rape honey. "Multifloral" honey comes from nectar collected from more than one type of flower.

Some honeys may have a mild taste, while other types possess a strong flavor. Some honey varietals (sunflower) are better used in baked goods than consumed raw.

Some shouldn't be used for baking, as they are delicacies (acacia, canola etc.) to be eaten straight from the jar.

Honeydew honeys are dark in color. Some of them are only popular amongst connoisseurs.

Is honey superior to table sugar?

I was quite surprised how much confusion is there about this topic when I tried to find out for myself how the sugars contained in honey are actually transformed into energy in our body.

You won't find too many sources where the layman can find clear and lucid information about the differences in how honey and table sugar deliver energy to our body.

There are all kinds of descriptions, but they miss the point and one is easily distracted by the Latin names of the sugar types and metabolic processes of breakdowns and transformations.

Due to this confusion, no wonder even some nutritionists say that honey is not superior to table sugar (sucrose) and it is only another "sweetener" of equal rank. But that doesn't stand up to scrutiny or personal experiences.

Well, let's try to make it a bit clearer.

Just having a quick look at the sugar types present in honey, we soon realize that there is a huge difference between honey and table sugar.

Honey is composed (up to 80% its weight) of three different types of "sugars" while table sugar is made up of only one type of sugar. Well, three is three times more than one, isn't it?

I have put sugars in quotation marks because actually the third type of carbohydrate compound of honey – oligosaccharides – chemically speaking are not regarded as sugars though they represent a group of 3-10 sugars joined together.

The following distinctions are important.

The main type of sugar in honey belongs to monosaccharides (called also simple sugars). They comprise 65-70% of the honey's weight and they are the most basic units of carbohydrates, which means they cannot be broken down further into simpler chemical compounds. So the simple sugars, glucose and fructose, in honey can be utilized by our body as soon as honey has been ingested.

Disaccharides – called also double sugars – are joined by a glycosidic bond which is a kind of covalent bond. They need to be broken down in the body to simple sugars so that they can be utilized. Table sugar, or sucrose, is a disaccharide. Actually this type of sugar is common in honey and table sugar, but while in refined table sugar it comprises the whole composition in honey it's only 0,5 to 5 % of its weight.

Oligosaccharides (actually not regarded as sugar!) are 3 to 10 simple sugars linked together by glycosodic bonds. They have been found to being able to re-establish the balance of the gut microbiota ecosystem.

Why are the sugar types in honey metabolized more easily?

There is a huge difference in how the sugars in honey are metabolized compared to table sugar. Table sugar, or sucrose, due to its disaccharide (double sugar) composition passes through the stomach without being broken down as the enzymes in the stomach aren't able to do this.

The breakdown of sucrose into its constituents, glucose and fructose, practically takes place first in the small intestine. The liver uses some enzymes to transform the molecules into glucose, which is then able to enter our bloodstream, from where it is absorbed by the body to refuel muscles, the brain and other organs.

In contrast to this, the bees have already done this work in honey by adding their enzymes to breakdown sucrose into two simple sugars, as mentioned before: fructose and glucose. These sugars are directly absorbed and the liver can do its job of transformation.

Honey contains an almost equal ratio of the simple sugars fructose and glucose – the exact ratio depends on the honey varietal. In 100 grams of honey there are about 35 grams of fructose and 35 grams of glucose, 0,5-5grams of disaccharides (like sucrose, maltose, isomaltose, maltulose, kojibiose and turanose) and about 3-4 grams of oligosaccharides like erlose, theanderose and panose.

A third type of carbohydrates – oligosaccharides – make honey a potential prebiotic, nourishing the intestinal microflora.

As we have seen the simple sugars, fructose and glucose, from the honey are easily absorbed already in the stomach.

The double sugars (sucrose, maltose etc.) in the honey will be digested the same way as table sugar would be, that means in the small intestine.

But in contrast to disaccharides, the oligosaccharides – the third type of "sugar" in honey- are not easily absorbed in the small intestine.

Oligosaccharides have to move into the large intestine to be digested. That also means they can serve as great sources of nutrients for our intestinal microflora.

Oligosaccharides are hydrolyzed (broken down) by the gut microbiota to produce short-chain fatty acids (acetate, lactate, etc), gases (carbon dioxide, methane etc.) and other metabolites.[12]

Studies show that oligosaccharides can reestablish the balance of the gut microbiota ecosystem. They can inhibit the growth and activity of harmful bacteria such as Staphylococcus, Proteus, Clostridium, Escherichia and Veillonella and they can help with the growth of Bifidobacteria and Lactobacilli in vitro.[13]

Though further research is needed in humans to examine the exact mechanisms, honey is increasingly being recognized as a potential prebiotic.[14]

And that was only comparing the sugar types of honey to table sugar, be it raw or refined. When making further comparisons, in refined table sugar you won't find enzymes, antioxidants, etc.

181 substances have been isolated in different honey varietals including 6 different vitamins, 12-14 minerals, 17 trace elements, 5 enzymes, 8 distinctive lipids, 18 different acids, 18 proteins (amino-acids), 18 bioflavonoids (antioxidants) and 26 aroma composites.

Probably it is no accident that every drop of honey – besides its sugars – is loaded with the above substances. Bees need instant and continuous energy (sugar) intake in the winter or when warming their brood. In both cases they have to regulate the temperature in the hive and keep it constant.[i] That's a difference between them and other insects. In contrast to other insects, bees are able to precisely regulate the temperature in the hive thanks to the energy gained from honey and become independent of the weather and temperature of the season or their environment. The worker bees will hatch from the brood in 21 days. The breeding time of other insects depends strongly on the outside temperatures.

Many of the almost two hundred compounds in honey are probably there for the survival of the bees. We don't yet know exactly how they help regulate the right absorption of sugars in honey, but they might have an important role and substantial impact on honey's health-giving properties in humans as well.

So far no experiment has been able to repeat the metabolic benefits of honey by simply mimicking its sugar composition.

---

i When overwintering, they keep a constant temperature of 12-25 °C (54-77°F)in their cluster. Then from spring to fall they keep 34.5-36 °C (94-96°F) in the brood so that the larvae develop continuously.

It seems that there are substances in honey that regulate the protein hormone[i] produced in the human liver which eases the uptake of glucose into muscle cells to be stored there as glycogen, resulting in lower sugar levels in our blood.

Honey is swiftly absorbed and transformed into glycogen in our liver. Thus glucose is removed from blood circulation and blood sugar levels are reduced so there is less demand for insulin release.

Composition, prebiotic and metabolic effects are those factors that differentiate honey from glucose, table sugar or HFCS.

What would taking two tablespoons of raw honey daily do for you?

When using honey in a smart and moderate way over a longer period it may help mouth and gut microbiome normalize. If one takes care for some other issues, like a lack of vitamins and minerals or make lifestyle changes, the probability of developing cavities – if you have any – will be reduced.[15]

It's been also found that the regular consumption of honey has positive influence on gastric ulcers, obesity, osteoporosis, all the chronic adrenalin-driven diseases, heart diseases, hypertension, type 2 diabetes, and dementia.[16]

Well, all these conditions won't change from one day to another from eating one or two tablespoons of raw honey each day, just as they didn't develop in a few days, but they are the consequences of a longer routine or other factors.

But, when thinking of lifestyle changes and implementing them as well, the right honey varietals or a blend of them can improve some of these conditions over time. Of course, excesses of the golden carbohydrate aren't good either and if used too much it can have adverse effects as well.

---

[i] Called Hepatic Insulin-sensitizing Substance (HISS)

How much sugar should I eat in a day?

No matter how the sugar industry argues that statistically it's not possible to show causation between added sugar consumption and chronic disease in humans – mostly because it is difficult to find large population groups not consuming added sugar to be the control groups – the excessive consumption of added sugar (sucrose) has been associated with the onset of diabetes, tooth decay, obesity, cardiovascular disease, dementia, certain cancers, non-alcoholic fatty liver disease etc.[17] [18]

In developed countries, an average individual eats about 33.1 kg (73lb) of sugar (sucrose) each year which is about 90 grams/day. That is over 360 food calories. In everyday language, we use calories for kcal. When talking about 360 calories in most of the cases we aren't talking about 0,360 kcal but about 360 kcal. Researchers measure energy in joules (J) or in its multiples (kJ).

The recent US dietary recommendation is similar to the WHO suggestion of a few years ago: people should limit their intake of added sugar to less than 10% of their daily calorie intake. The WHO even suggests, if possible, to go below 5%. Some European countries also suggests 5% or about 25-30 grams.

Thus, women should consume between 100-200 kcal (25-50 grams) of free sugar per day; while men should consume: 130-260 kcal (32.5-65 grams) of free sugar per day.

If we take a look at the average amount of sugar added to food in western society, 25-65 grams is actually not very much and it is exhausted very quickly with a can of soda, some chocolates, ice cream or biscuits: a can of soda (355 mL-12 US fl. oz.) already contains 39 grams.

How much honey should I consume?

Some therapists use honey in relatively large amounts (250-300 grams a day). Using honey in such a high amount for curing or therapeutical purposes can be justified, but unless you are a specialist or you are under controlled circumstances in a clinic, I'd rather say take care with the intake of such high amounts of carbohydrates.

Considering the aforementioned recommendations, we would say that you can eat 20% more honey than the previous recommendations for free sugar, as sugar is about 80% of honey's weight: women: 30-60 grams and men 39-78 grams of honey a day – when not eating other sugar-containing food or sweets. The remaining 17-19% of the honey is water and 0.5-1 % minerals, enzymes, amino acids, proteins and vitamins which practically doesn't provide any calories or just a negligible amount.

Honey only contains 0.5-to 5 percent disaccharides (sucrose) that are metabolized differently than simple sugars.

The main "sweet" carbohydrate components of honey are monosaccharides (simple sugars) and in smaller amounts oligosaccharides 2-5% (not even regarded as sugars!).

That means if you eat 20% more honey than the daily recommendation in grams for added or free sugar – let's take the maximum of our calculation for women: 60 gram a day – you'll only take in 0.3 to 3 grams of sucrose and 15-20 grams fructose and 15-20 grams glucose and about 1-5 grams oligosaccharides.

Well, two tablespoons of honey a day (2x22-28 grams) one tablespoon in the morning, and one at bedtime, it is a minimum if one wants to profit from the beneficial effects of honey (pure, raw and not adulterated!) – improving metabolic stress caused insomnia, or reducing blood sugar levels, improving the immune system, strengthening or reestablishing the balance of the gut microbiota, etc.

What about teaspoons and tablespoons?

In some cases it's good to know how much honey or sugar is on your spoon. But a tablespoon of crystallized honey is more than a tablespoon of liquid honey, as you'll take more of it from the jar at once and liquid honey will flow off your tablespoon.

If it's important to you, for one reason or another, to know exactly how much honey you consume, weigh how much honey your spoons can hold, both from crystallized honey and liquid honey.

One tablespoon of honey is about 22-28 gr (66-85kcal) while a teaspoon of honey is about 7-11 grams (24-33kcal), whereas a tablespoon of sugar weighs 13-16g (52-64kcal) and a teaspoon of sugar is about 4-6g (16-24kcal).

Personally, I don't worry too much about it, I just count how many tablespoons of honey I have consumed in a day, maximum 3-4. I usually don't exceed that amount. If I eat other carbohydrate-rich food like potatoes, rice, fruits, then I take care not to eat more than one or two tablespoons of honey a day. If I want to loose some weight I only take my one tablespoon of honey at bedtime.

The smart use of honey

As you'll see in the honey varietal section of this book, different honeys contain different amounts of immunostimulating and antimicrobial factors, different ratios of glucose/fructose or different amount of oligosaccharides, etc.

In order to experience all the benefits of honey in my daily honey consumption, I eat at least two types of honey. At bedtime I mostly ingest less acidic honeys, such as canola (rape) or chestnut honey. In the morning I take acacia and during the day some other types we have in our pantry, such as sunflower, linden etc.

When I see that there are infections in my surroundings, in my family or at the school where I teach, I eat honey with turmeric and black pepper or honey with propolis (see in *Honey recipe,* page 109) for a few days and take more care with the hygiene of my mouth, nose and throat.

An important aspect of my honey consumption in the morning and evening is that after I have ingested honey I don't eat or drink anything else for half an hour. Thus I let the honey provide its effects.

During the day I use honey as a sweetener in coffee and tea, taking care not to exceed the total daily amount of 3-4 tablespoons of honey.

I have to add that I don't drink soft drinks or soda or eat food containing added sugar or HFCS. In my experience, it's best to remove these from our diet.

Teaching the brain to give up sugar-rich food and drinks

It's not easy to stop consuming foods and drinks with added sugar if it is an established habit. Our brain, probably stimulated by some bacteria of our microbiota, longs for sucrose as an important and easily available source of energy. We all get used to this as this source of energy is omnipresent and offered to us everywhere in seducing and delicious forms. Maybe we can only talk about addiction in a few cases, as it is possible to give it up. If we teach our brain that there is another much healthier source of energy we'll be able to give it up.

Many people have succeeded in giving up sugar and sugar-containing food and drinks by taking a teaspoon of honey each time they have a longing for chocolate, biscuits, soft drinks etc.

In the recipe section you'll find some delicacies made of honey. Preparing and using them is an option, but raw honey will also do the trick when taking it to give up sugar.

A parallel measure to eating honey whenever one longs for sugary food and soft drinks is to re-establish one's gut microbiota with pre- and probiotics.

Honey helps with this as well, as the oligosaccharides provide nutrients to our gut bacteria. But you can also improve it by eating healthy foods, such as legumes, fruits, salads, fish and other healthy meat, avoiding or reducing starch.

Glycemic indexes of some honey varietals:

Glycemic index is useful for quantifying the relative rapidity with which the body breaks down carbohydrates. That means honey glycemic index tells how quickly, or slowly, its sugars are turned into blood glucose.

Glycemic index can be used to assess the insulin response burden of a food. A food has a low GI if it is 55 or less; mid-range GI if 56 to 69, high GI if 70 or more.[19]

> *The good news is that the glycemic index of honey varies between 32 and 64, which is lower than sugar – white or brown – at 65.*

The GI varies with the level of fructose – the more fructose, the lower the GI.[20] Acacia 34, Chestnut, linden and heather honey between 49-55,
Rapeseed honey 64, Honey dew 89.

Is honey for people with diabetes?

If you have diabetes (type 1, 1,5 or 2) consult your physician or a specialist before making dietary changes.

Eating refined table sugar and HFCS increases insulin levels in your blood and eventually leads to insulin resistance. But that's not the case with honey, given we consume it moderately.[21]

Insulin is produced by our pancreas and helps cells in our body to take up sugar for energy. As sugar cannot enter our cells directly, insulin attaches to and signals cells to absorb it from the blood circulation. Insulin may be also described as a "key" that unlocks the cells which then let sugars enter.

Having more sugar in the body than needed, insulin helps store it in our liver.

Insulin is important because it balances out blood sugar levels. If blood sugar levels rise, more insulin will be secreted by beta cells of the pancreatic islets.

If someone has diabetes, it means his or her body does not produce enough insulin or his or her cells are resistant to insulin.

There are several ongoing and new research projects regarding the absorption of sugars in honey. You may share and discuss these results with your physician or nutritionist (see in *Why are the sugar types in honey metabolized more easily?*, *page 60*).

Of course, most of the research is limited to small groups or, in some cases, in vitro and haven't been analyzed with large groups or with large control groups. That might prevent the nutritionist from advising you to eat honey.

In most cases physicians and nutritionists allow patients with diabetes to eat fruits or legumes in moderate amounts. Actually a tablespoon of honey does not contain more sugar than a small cup of fruit, or an apple.

In addition, the sugars in honey (if the honey is raw, pure, ripe and not adulterated) are metabolized differently.

There is research of the Honey Tolerance Test (similar to the Glucose Tolerance Test) available that confirms that ingesting honey results in lower blood sugar levels.[22]

After the consumption of honey, at 60 and 90 minutes, test results show a 20 and 40 mg% lower blood sugar level than in the glucose and sucrose tests.

It seems that there are substances in honey which are believed to act as regulators of the protein hormone produced in the liver, called hepatic insulin-sensitizing substance (HISS) which eases the uptake of glucose into muscle cells to be stored there as glycogen resulting in lower sugar levels in our blood.

> *Honey is swiftly absorbed and transformed into glycogen in our liver. Thus glucose is removed from blood circulation and blood sugar levels are reduced and there is less demand for insulin release.*

It must also be mentioned that honey is able to increase the quantity of good bacteria in the intestines. Some of these have been associated with positive effects in diabetics, helping with glucose control and regulating insulin function.[23]

Paradoxically, adding honey to one's diet, along with removing most added sugar/HFCS/starch, could be a treatment for type 2 diabetes.[24][25][26]

But patients with type 1 diabetes have also presented positive effects from the long-term intake of honey.[27][28]

Honey varietals with low GI are recommended for diabetics (type 2) as well.

Some therapists say that honey is a good choice for diabetics because of its ratio of 1:1 fructose – glucose.

Ron Fessenden says in his book, *The New Honey Revolution: Restoring the Health of Future Generations*, that a 1:1 ratio of fructose and glucose is entirely transformed by the liver into glycogen, and there will be no other sugars left to enter the blood. "This perfect ratio, along with flavonoids and all the others constituents of honey, some of them as yet not identified, recommend it for the use of diabetics, even leading to improvements of their condition."

Is honey for vegans?

Some vegans are of the opinion that honey is not ethical to consume as beekeepers exploit their colonies for profit. While, this may be true for industrial beekeeping, but it is not true for all beekeepers. As a small-scale beekeeper, I can state that I and most of my colleagues help our bees and even though we may take the surplus of the honey from the hive, we leave more than enough for the bees. Besides this, when the bees cannot collect nectar, which has happened a few times in recent years due to climate change, we feed the bees for survival.

Beekeepers contribute to maintaining colonies near agricultural fields, in orchards and gardens so that the bees can accomplish the needful pollination.

In these areas, due to some chemicals used in agriculture or parasites spread in the last 30-40 years (like the varroa mite), bees would not survive without the help of the beekeepers.

If it matters to you that bees are kept in a bee-friendly way you may ask the beekeeper at the market directly. It'd be a pity not to consume or use honey, this healing and delicious gift of the bees.

Warnings:

Don't eat too much honey!
When experiencing the benefits of honey one may throw caution to the wind and consume large amounts of honey. Don't do that. Enjoy honey and life by being moderate, like a connoisseur. You may have read this warning before in this book, but I repeat it, as it is actually a warning to myself as well!

Why shouldn't infants under a year old eat honey?
Don't give honey to babies under one year. There is a very small chance, but honey can contain inactive spores of a bacterium that may

multiply in infants' immature guts and which is responsible for botulism food poisoning (Clostridium botulinum). Healthy adults don't get sick from it.

Summary

- The honey is ready when most of the water has been dried out of the nectar by the bees and less than 18-19% remains.

- Honey is primarily classified by the type of plant the nectar or honeydew was collected from: acacia honey, pine honey etc.

- In 100 grams of honey there are about 35 grams of fructose and 35 grams of glucose, 0,5-5grams of and about 3-4 grams of oligosaccharides.

- 181 substances have been isolated in different honey varietals (vitamins, minerals, trace elements, enzymes, distinctive lipids, acids, proteins, bioflavonoids (antioxidants) respectively aroma composites.

- Composition, prebiotic and metabolic effects are those factors that differentiate honey profoundly from glucose, table sugar or HFCS.

- The regular consumption of honey has positive influence on gastric ulcers, obesity, osteoporosis, all the chronic adrenalin-driven diseases, heart diseases, hypertension, type 2 diabetes and dementias.

- Two tablespoons of honey a day it is a minimum if one wants to profit from the beneficial effects of honey (pure, raw and not adulterated honey!)

- The glycemic index of honey varies between 32 and 64, which is lower than sugar – white or brown – at 65.

- Honey is swiftly absorbed and transformed into glycogen in our liver and there is less demand for insulin release.

- Enjoy honey by being moderate!

- Don't give honey to babies under one year!

5. DIFFERENT FORMS OF THE HONEY

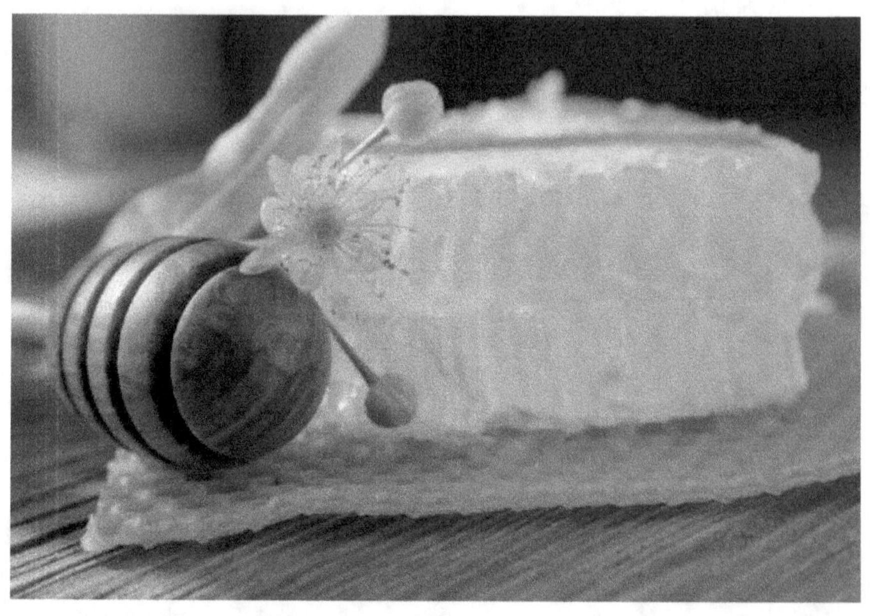

In this section you'll learn:

- The differences between raw, pasteurized, organic, blended, creamed and comb honey;

- When honey is ripe;

- How to decrystallize honey without damaging its important constituents;

Raw vs pasteurized honey

In supermarkets most of the honey has been heated briefly at 60°C (140° F) and then cooled. In order to look clearer and more appealing on the shelf, it will be also filtered by the manufacturer. This „pasteurization" prevents the honey from fermenting and slows down its crystallization. But it also reduces its enzymes and antioxidants. Moreover heat produces toxic HMF (Hydroximethylfurfural) in honey.

That's why it is recommended to buy honey from a beekeeper you know well or from shops where you can be assured that the honey you are buying hasn't been heated or filtered.

Ripe honey vs dried honey

Honey is ripe when it contains about 17-19% water. That also indicates that the bees have regurgitated it many times and added their enzymes to the nectar, so that most of the sucrose is cleaved into two basic simple sugars, glucose and fructose, which can be easily absorbed by our body.

Sometimes the beekeeper extracts honey before this process is finished. The honey is then unripe. That is not only bad for the consistency or storability of the honey – it remains liquid – but it means that the sucrose hasn't been cleaved properly by the bees.

A few beekeepers do this deliberately and dry the extracted unripe honey in special dryers to evaporate the excess water. Thus the consistency, storability and shelf life of the honey may be okay, but the sucrose content will be much higher and the substances added by the bees much lower than expected in honey. For this reason "dried honey" cannot be considered honey!

Organic honey?

Honey bees fly up to 3-4 kilometers (2-3miles) to collect nectar, which it makes impossible to determine whether they have only visited flowers of organically produced plants. That's why the label "organic honey" only gives information on whether the honey in the jar was produced by a beekeeper using bee friendly methods or only organic acids and medicine against some bee parasites and pests.

Blended honey

Blended honey means that multiple sources of honey have been mixed.

They may come from different countries as well. Beekeepers in the EU hope not only for better regulation of the honey standards, but also for its labelling, as at the moment only a ridiculous description of the origins of the honey is required: "A blend from EU and non-EU countries". Which could even mean that it comes from the Moon!

Comb Honey

In comb honey, the honey is still enclosed within its original hexagonal-shaped beeswax cells which we call honeycomb. It is consumed as produced by honey bees.

It's very delicious and its flavor differs a bit from extracted raw honey as you can enjoy the flavor and enzymes of the beeswax in it as well. I know people who are great fans of it and are only willing to eat comb honey and turn me down when I offer them extracted honey.

You may eat some beeswax when eating comb honey but beware not all its components are digestible. So it is better to spit it out.

Some naturopath healers ascribe healing and spiritual power to the hexagonal cells and recommend comb honey, of course in very small amounts, in therapies.

A great advantage of comb honey is that it has not been filtered or processed.

As not every beekeeper produces it, comb honey is a premium delicacy with a relatively high price.

A definite disadvantage of comb honey, as I can confirm, is that it is very difficult to be moderate about eating it once you have it in your kitchen.

Crystalized honey vs. sugar syrup – checking adulteration

Some people think honey crystallizes because the beekeeper has put sugar in it.

Actually, crystallization occurs naturally in honey.

Crystallization of honey helps preserve the quality of its nutrients. It happens because honey contains a huge amount of sugar dissolved in a relative small amount of water. At least 77-80% of the carbohydrates are dissolved in less than 18-19% water. This is more sugar than can normally stay in solute form and crystals start to form over time.

There are honeys which form fine and smooth crystals over a short period (i.e. rapeseed honey) and others (i.e. sunflower) which form large crystals over a longer period.

Whether a honey forms finer or larger crystals depends on the fructose and glucose ratio in it. While fructose remains dissolved more easily, glucose possesses lower solubility.

The more glucose the honey contains, the more quickly it crystallizes.

More rapidly crystallized honey contains finer, smoother crystals.

Creamed honey also called spun honey

In creamed honey the large number of small crystals hinders the formation of larger ones

The beekeeper can "grind" the crystals and make excellent creamed honey by stirring the honey with the right tool (a kind of sterile "paint" stirrer) each day for a few minutes when the crystallization process starts.

You can create creamed honey by simply putting it into the fridge for a while and then returning it at room temperature. Though this does not work for all types of honey, it works well with acacia.

Be aware that creamed honey from large manufacturers is produced by heating the honey, which can lead to nutritional losses.

When buying local creamed honey, ask the beekeeper, how it was made.

See how you can make your home made creamed honey at the recipe section.

Decrystallization

If you prefer liquid honey you can easily decrystallize it by putting the glass jar (without a lid) of crystallized honey into a pot with water that comes ½ to ⅔ up the sides of the jar.

Heat the water to a warm temperature which is still comfortable for your hands. Maintain steady heat 40-45°C (104°-115°F).

Stir the honey every few minutes until the honey is once again smooth and runny.

If the honey is overheated, some of the important enzymes and other nutrients are destroyed.

Summary

- The label "organic honey" only gives information on whether the honey was produced by a beekeeper using organic acids or organic treatments against some bee parasites and pests.

- Blended honey means that multiple sources of honey have been mixed.

- A great advantage of comb honey is that it has not been filtered or processed.

- Crystallization occurs naturally in honey.

- There are honey varietals which form fine and smooth crystals over a short period (e.g. rapeseed honey) and others which form large crystals over a longer period (e.g. sunflower).

- The more glucose the honey contains, the more quickly it crystallizes.

- In creamed honey the large number of small crystals hinders the formation of larger ones.

- If you prefer liquid honey you can easily decrystallize it.

6. HONEY VARIETALS – TASTE THEM ALL!

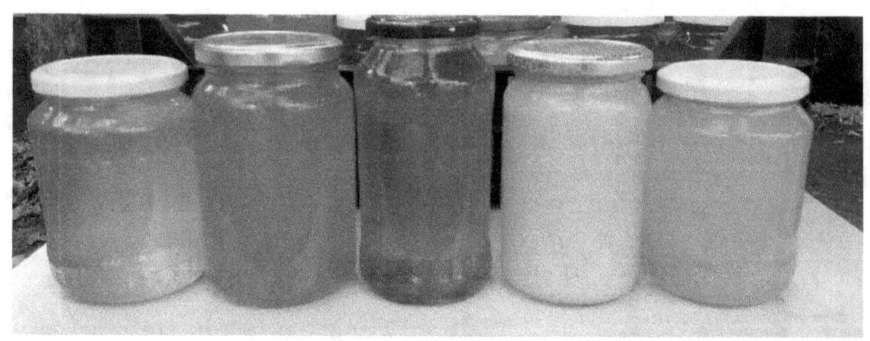

In this section you'll learn:

- Why you should discover your local honey varietals;

- Some of my local honey varietals;

- "Exotic" and exclusive honey varietals

- Why to taste honey whenever you have the chance;

Each honey varietal has got its own personality

Through the ratio of its compounds, the honey bears the characteristics of the landscape and season.

No honey varietal is the same in subsequent years, just as wine can have nuances differing from the previous year. Before each extraction I can hardly wait to find out how the honey will taste.

The first taste of freshly extracted honey is a special and revered moment, a kind of ritual for my family and me.

There are more than 300 honey varietals. There is a lack of space to describe them all here and it wouldn't add much either. The best is anyway to find out about your local honeys is by asking beekeepers in your area or on the market.

It is also amazing to "collect" honey flavors when traveling. You may try local honeys wherever you are. It's surprising what kinds of honeys exist depending on the herbal characteristics of a certain region.

I'll describe here the most common characteristics of my local types of honey that I extract from my hives and which I have the most experience with in using as remedies or as "sweetener".

I'll also touch upon some honey varietals that are not typical to my region but that are worth tasting or using if you get the chance. Some of them are real rarities and you cannot buy them in shops, only wait for them to cross your path or you are there when they are harvested.

Canola honey

Let's start with my favorite honey, also called by the ugly name "rape honey". It comes from the rapeseed nectar, from those beautiful yellow blooming fields (Brassica napus) in spring. You can see them all over North America or Central and Eastern Europe.

It is my favorite honey varietal for at least three reasons.

> *1. It has "low" acidity. If you have stomach issues or re-flux you'll love canola honey, it's actually the only type of honey that soothes stomach pain caused by too much acid or ulcers.*

2. Its taste is excellent, It's like marzipan. You can use it as the base for some sweets I will recommend here instead of chocolates and against stomach pain in the recipe section (see at *Honey recipes*)!

3. It has a lovely color and consistency. It crystallizes very rapidly, which means it has a high glucose and a lower fructose content. Canola honey only stays runny for 5-7 days after being extracted. It has very fine crystals. I am amazed at its color as well. It's white to clear creamy. When it is pure, as the bees didn't collect other different nectars, it is so white that you'd confuse it with fat.

Though it has a relative high glycemic index among the honey types – GI 64 – it doesn't exceed that of refined sugar and, interestingly, studies say that after eating canola honey, the fructose level in blood doesn't rise (or it is just similar) as after eating acacia honey (GI of acacia 35-44). Studies suggest fructose metabolism may be repressed by unidentified substances in the canola honey.[29]

This suggests that even if the GI of canola honey is relatively high, it's wrong to deny it to diabetics. As we have seen earlier in this book small amounts of honey with a 50-50% glucose/fructose ratio are healthy for type 2 diabetics.

Canola honey has its drawbacks as well. There are countries (e.g. US) where they use genetically modified rapeseed crops, so if you are determined not to consume genetically modified food you have to take care where this variety of honey comes from.

The immunostimulating effect of canola honey is rather low, but it depends on when the honey was harvested and how much albumin1 it contains. When this honey comes from the hive when there are already queen larvae to be fed by worker bees, canola honey will have higher doses of this immunostimulating enzyme.

Its peroxide and non-peroxide activity, compared to other honeys, is considered intermediate.

In folks medicine it is recommended for peptic ulcers, kidney disease and to lower cholesterol.

Acacia Honey

It has a light amber color. It's very sweet with a pure floral taste.

Acacia honey is very popular as it has high fructose and low glucose concentrations and for this reason it crystallizes only slowly. It is made of black locust tree blossoms, and not from real acacia.

Its scientific name is Robinia pseudocacia: False acacia!

Once I forgot a container of acacia honey in my bee shed and in the spring I was astonished when I found it and initially thought that the winter hadn't done it any good.

I had never seen crystallized acacia honey before. Thanks to its popularity in my family we never keep it too long in our pantry.

After taking it into the kitchen it became "creamed" in one day. It was the most delicious creamed honey I have ever tasted. Since then I have taken to putting some jars of acacia honey into the fridge for a while to become creamed.

You can make creamed honey out of it without grinding the crystals. Most diabetics can also enjoy it in small amounts without any problems as it has a very low Glycemic Index which is about 35.

It's said that the antioxidants of acacia honey help fight heart disease and even some forms of cancer.

To my knowledge there is no scientific evidence for that.

On the other hand, it is proven that acacia honey is very effective against bacteria as it slowly releases hydrogen peroxide.

We have seen that releasing hydrogen peroxide when honey absorbs free water from the surroundings is important in how honey works against pathogens.

For that reason I use acacia in the recipes given in this book for homemade remedies

The immunostimulating effects of acacia may be intermediate as it contains about 0,010% apalbumin 1.

Therapeutical uses (not researched but used in folk medicine!):

- for complaints of asthma, in issues of the stomach, intestines, liver and kidney;
- it relieves apnea,
- It increases bile acid.
- It calms the nervous system (best honey to be taken before bedtime.)
- Sweetener for people with Diabetes 2.

Chestnut honey

Its color is dark to very dark. It's rather bitter with a low acidity of about pH 4. Due to its high fructose and low glucose content, this honey varietal remains for a long time in a liquid state.

Chestnut honey is the main ingredient in Vivamel (a medical honey used for treating wounds).

A set of analyses confirmed that chestnut honey is very effective for wound healing.[30]

It has about 40% fructose and about 28% glucose and a low GI between 49 and 55.

It's collected from Sweet Chestnut (Castanea sativa). It is a very good nectar and pollen source for bees, but it also offers some honeydew, produced by some insects that parasitize on it like Myzocallis castanicola, Rhynchota Homoptera, Lachnus roboris L. etc.

Bees also collect the honeydew secreted by these insects on the tree's bark.

Its immunostimulating effect is rather high as it has a high apalbumin1 content, one of the highest amongst the spring honeys.

This honey varietal has average to high peroxide and non-peroxide activity, which means its antibacterial effect has a very good range.

It has gastroprotective properties.

Linden(EU)- basswood(US) or Lime (UK) honey

Its color ranges from pale yellow to darker yellow. Its taste is very sweet having a touch of bitterness and astringency. It is considered an acidic honey.

It contains an almost equal ratio of fructose and glucose. It starts crystallizing 3-4 months after being extracted.

Linden honey:

• is rich in maltose (7-8%) which is beneficial to our digestive system.

• compared to other honeys, it has a great number of vitamins and macronutrients, (Vitamin B1, B2, B5, B6), nicotinic acid, Vitamin H, zinc, cobalt, calcium, sulfur, potassium, copper, iodine, phosphorus, chlorine, magnesium, etc.)

• organic and inorganic acids like lactic, gluconic, citric, linolenic acid, oxalic acid, phosphoric acid etc.

Of course honey can never be the principal source of these vitamins and macronutrients, as in fact these are present in very low amounts in the honey.

Thanks to its very rich content of enzymes and antioxidants linden honey is recommended for preventing tonsillitis and controlling the inflammation of respiratory organs and it is a good choice for digestive problems or for gastritis and colitis.

It eases the discharge of the mucus from the nose and throat. It has laxative and diuretic effects.

For this reasons the use of linden honey is indicated for only a limited time.

Personally, when taking it in the winter and seasonal flu infection periods, I really like its special astringent taste and its effect against colds is obvious. But after a maximum of a week I find it nauseating and I don't long for it.

Linden honey is contraindicated:

• in the last semester of pregnancy because some of its constituents may thin the blood and increase the risk of hemorrhage after birth.

• for people with acute heart failure, anemia (as it blocks the absorption of iron)

• for drivers: it can cause sleepiness.

Sunflower honey

It is a summer honey varietal. It has a bright, medium yellow color. I'd say it smells and tastes "fruity". It's not as sweet as acacia and it lacks any bitterness.

It's important to know that in contrast to canola (rapeseed honey), it is highly acidic.

I remember when I first extracted sunflower honey it caused me stomach pain. You should know that most beekeepers find extracting honey is a good opportunity to overeat, as that's the moment when the fresh golden miracle tastes most delicious. It still contains all the flavors and aromas put in by Mother Nature and the bees. Unfortunately many of these will evaporate with time. From this perspective, it isn't any wonder that I got stomachache from it.

By the way that's another reason why I keep telling you, find your local beekeepers and their honey. You could even offer to help with honey harvest; help is always wanted in an apiary. Well, I don't know whether they will welcome your proposal, but if so, it would be the experience of a lifetime. Beware: don't overeat the honey.

Sunflower honey is mostly used for baking, and manufacturers mix it into other "inferior" honeys to improve them. But of course, it also has its beneficial effects just like other honey varietals.

It crystalizes with raw crystals. Making it creamy changes its color to a lighter yellow than when crystallized normally. To me, creamed sunflower honey seems to be less acidic then its liquid version.

Sunflower honey is very rich in pollen and it's a very good resource for bees in wintertime. My grandfather believed that extracting sunflower honey is extremely important as it crystallizes relatively quickly with raw crystals and the bees cannot digest it during the winter. But since then it's turned out that it is one of the best overwintering honeys for the bees.

The protein-rich pollen in sunflower honey left for the bees for overwintering helps them to start breeding at a time when there is no other pollen or nectar resource yet in the environment.

„Exotic" honey varietals

The following honey varietals aren't available in my region. I have tasted some (Manuka honey, forest honey, buckwheat honey, thyme) when traveling and there are some I'm still waiting to come across (Bashkir honey, heather honey, Anzer honey). But remember, each region has its own "famous" honey varietals with high curative properties. You may ask around and search for them whenever you are travelling.

Manuka honey

It has antimicrobial properties and it's able to increase the efficacy of antibiotic drugs.

Manuka honey contains 100 to1000 times the natural concentration of MGO (methylglyoxal) – a powerful antibacterial agent- of other honeys. Manuka honey, when real and containing the correct amount of MGO, is a very expensive bee product (at the moment 1 kg is about 450-500 dollars). If you want to use it, make sure you buy the real thing. Cheap Manuka honey may be adulterated or contain only a small amount of MGO. Look for UMF on the label, which is a grade granted by the Unique Manuka Factor Honey Association of New Zealand and represents a standard of quality.

Heather honey

It is a reddish-brown amber honey with high fructose levels made from *Calluna vulgaris*. In Britain, it is appreciated as the "Rolls Royce" of honeys by connoisseurs.

Both heather and manuka honeys are thixotropic, which is to say they are "gel-like" when standing still. When stirred or agitated they turn liquid again.

The extraction of heather honey from the comb is difficult as its viscosity is very high.

Thyme honey

It is a light amber to amber honey collected from *Thymus vulgaris*. It has a very strong, intense aroma with resinous, savory flavors. It crystallizes in a short time, just as canola honey does, into medium or fine grains.

If you've ever enjoyed the fragrance of thyme in the mountains, you'll love this honey, too. But it is rather acidic and people with re-flux should consume it with care.

Anzer honey

It is polyfloral honey varietal harvested at high altitude on the Anzer Plateau in the Black Seas region of Turkey. It's believed to have innumerable benefits, like treating pharyngitis, tonsillitis, ulcers, preventing prostate issues, increasing sexual power, supporting growth, treating diarrhea, improving cardiac function etc. Its price starts at 300 dollars a kilo and goes up to 1000 dollars.

Bashkir honey

Some experts affirm that its taste and curative properties have *no equivalents in the world.*

This honey varietal is made by the Burzyan wild-hive bees, belonging to the European black bee, *Apis mellifera mellifera,* at high altitudes in the Southern Urals in the Republic of Baschkortostan, Russia.

These honeybees are adapted to survive the long, cold winters, sometimes even -45°, -50°C (-49°, -58°F).

The enzymes the Burzyan bees add to the nectar may be slightly different than the enzymes other honey bees add and probably that's what makes the difference.

Linden is the main floral source in this honey, but it's considered a multifloral honey as the bees mix in other regional nectars as well. It is one of the most expensive honey varietals in the world.

Summary

- There are more than 300 honey varietals.

- Canola honey soothes stomach pain caused by too much acid or ulcers. It's like "marzipan". You can use it as the base for some sweets It crystallizes very rapidly.

- Acacia Honey slowly releases hydrogen peroxide. It stays liquid for longer time at room temperature.

- Chestnut honey is rather bitter with a "low" acidity of about pH 4. It has gastro-protective properties.

- Linden(EU)- basswood(US) or lime(UK) honey is recommended for preventing tonsillitis and controlling the inflammation of respiratory organs and it is a good choice for digestive problems or for gastritis, colitis. It is contraindicated in certain cases.

- Sunflower honey smells and tastes "fruity". It is acidic.

- Each region has its own "famous" honey varietals with high curative properties. You should ask around and search for them whenever you travel.

7. HOW HONEY WORKS FOR OUR HEALTH

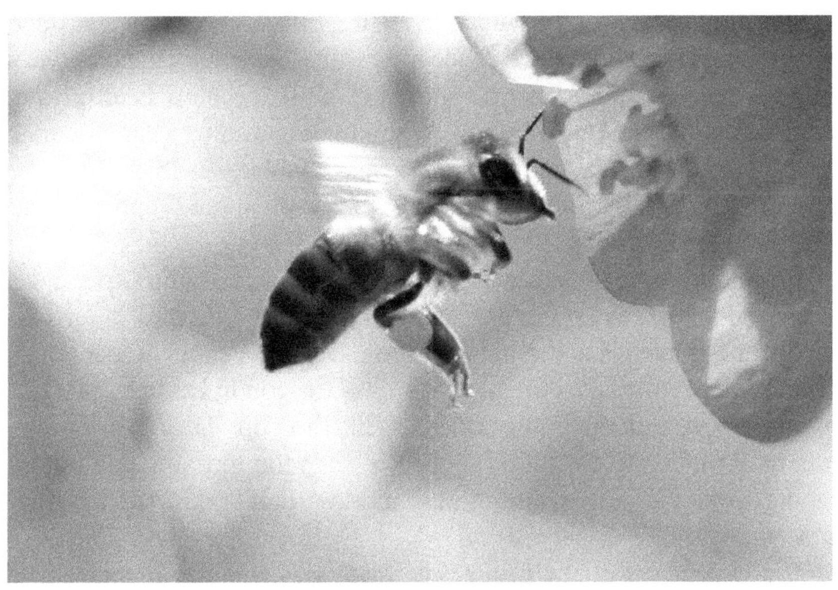

In this section you'll learn:

- What constituents of honey account for its healing power;

- How to use honey for injuries, colds, stomach pain, insomnia, obesity;

- Why it is advised to eat some honey when consuming alcohol;

- A recipe for massage oil with honey;

The secret of health?

As I'm a schoolteacher three times a year I have to regularly visit the doctor for an overall check-up. They take blood tests, measure my BMI (Body Mass Index), blood pressure, pulse, check my heart and lungs etc. When some doctors see my results, especially the blood test results they ask me what I do for my overall "perfect" health, what kind of exercises I do and so on. When I tell them that I eat moderate amounts of honey regularly, one tablespoon, about 22-28 grams in the morning and one before going to bed, they look at me skeptically and ask about other things as well.

Of course, there are other measures I take, I've learnt by experience, sometimes painful experience, which may have a serious impact on my overall physical and mind condition. But you cannot talk about all that in the few minutes the physician has for you in his busy practice with waiting patients in the corridor. But I'm convinced that the regular and moderate consumption of honey in the morning and before going to bed is one of the most important habits that supports my "good health".

I hasten to add that I'm not free from all health problems. Some issues are waiting for solutions (i.e. periodontitis and backache after handling my hives).

Honey can be immunostimulating and certain compounds of it are antimicrobial. Honey works multifactorially and that seems to be the key to its healing nature.

Immunostimulating effect

Apalbumin 1, is a compound found in royal jelly and it is present in some honey types as well. It has shown immunostimulating properties.[31] Apalbumin is present in certain honey varietals in different quantities. According to a study, its quantity decreases in the following order: chestnut 0.029%, dandelion 0.014%, acacia 0.011%; linden 0.010%; rape 0.010%; saccharose syrup honey contains only 0.001% apalbumin 1.[32]

Well, as a beekeeper I think this single study cannot really determine the right order or amount of apalbumin in different honey varietals. It's obvious that the above plants all bloom in the spring, in the season when bees feed the queen larvae (from the middle of spring till midsummer). It probably gets into the nectar when the mandibular gland of the bees is the most active and at the same time a lot of nectar comes into the hive. The most apalbumin1 will be in honey when the secretion of the bee's gland is at its peak.

Another important compound is kynurenic acid (KYNA) – mainly present in chestnut honey. KYNA is a metabolite of tryptophan and in animal experiments it exerts a number of positive actions: anti-inflammatory and antioxidative activity. KYNA inhibits the synthesis of pro-inflammatory cytokines and probably protects tissues from oxidative damage.[33]

The content of KYNA in chestnut honey is exceptionally high and that's why this honey varietal can be an important source of dietary KYNA.[34] Chestnut honey is the main ingredient of Vivamel, a medical honey product used for wound treatment.

Antimicrobial effects of honey

Let's have a look at the different healing compounds and mechanisms of honey. This "list" cannot be exhaustive as there are still many antimicrobial and immunostimulating effects of honey, which have not been elucidated, but hopefully will be added to in the future.

1.The most important compound in honey responsible for healing and prevention is an enzyme called glucose oxidase. It breaks down glucose sugars. When there is free water available in the surroundings it produces hydrogen peroxide which is a kind of bleach with an anti-spoiling nature.

Honey contains about 75-80% of sugar and there is very little – only 17-19% – water in it. Thus honey is likely to take up water from its surroundings. That means when honey is being rubbed on the skin or injuries it takes water from there, when eaten it takes water from the digestive system.

2. Another antimicrobial compound in honey is a peptide called Bee Defensin1. For a long time it was thought to be found exclusively in Royal Jelly (food produced by the worker bees for the Queen larvae), but scientists discovered it in honey as well.

> *3. The "healing" property of honey is due to its acidity as well. The pH of honey is approximately 3.5. Most pathogens can't handle this environment. But don't think honey is sterile, it may contain some spores.*

4. The compound called Methylglyoxal (MGO) is a powerful antibacterial agent. Unfortunately, it's only been found naturally in Manuka honey from New Zealand. MGO is making Manuka honey a potentially topical salve in clinical honey treatments, such as Medi-Honey.[35]

But precaution is needed when consuming it. Research indicates that MGO contributes to increased oxidative stress within body cells due to its rapid metabolism into advanced glycation end products. As MGO inhibits insulin it may be one cause of diabetes.[36]

It is believed[37] that MGO in most honey varietals (except Manuka honey containing it naturally) comes about when honey is heated. [i]

For this reasons overheated honey and manuka honey need to be used with precaution, especially by diabetics.

---

[i] In Europe, spot-checking of import honey at the border and local honey in shops prevents those with high amounts of HMF (Hydroxymethylfurfural) – an indicator for overheating – to enter the EU-countries or are banned from the shelves.

HOW TO USE HONEY FOR PREVENTION AND CURE

As mentioned earlier, therapists may use honey in relatively large amounts (250-300 grams a day). Using honey in such a high amount for curative or therapeutical purposes can be justified, but unless you are a specialist or you are under controlled circumstances in a clinic, I'd rather say take care with the intake of such high amounts of carbohydrates. Of course, if you wish, and your health allows it, you may experiment with the intake of large amounts of honey. But be sure to monitor yourself with observations, or if you have the chance, with some laboratory analyses as well.

When I am taking preventive measures against some pathogens, I eat very little sugar or food containing sugar and starch or even leave them out altogether. Depending on the gravity of the situation, I consider reducing my honey consumption as well.

I use our local honey varietals: linden (called also lime or basswood), acacia, chestnut, canola (rapeseed), sunflower, multiflora honey etc.

Honey for injuries and burns

Mild to mid-range injuries and second-degree burns seem to heal 4-5 days earlier when putting honey on them than with clinically used Silver sulfadiazine.[38]

One of my beekeeper colleagues suffered a grave accident with his motorcycle. His doctor told him his injury would take a long time to heal. The physician was quite astonished when the beekeeper showed up healed injuries much earlier than expected. He used honey on his injuries!

To be sure of the results we use Vivamel or Medihoney. In case of a grave injury/burn, a doctor is to be consulted, as in these cases special measures need to be taken.

Method:

First the injury or cut needs to be disinfected, then honey can be rubbed on it. With a second degree-burn, run cold water on it first then pure and germ free honey can be applied. If needed in order to protect the injury and not to smear everything with honey, one may put some bandages on it too and change them each day.

Honey for chronic diseases?

There are claims that honey cures asthma, arthritis, anemia or heart problems.

Honey can be a part of a therapy, but when being treated for chronic diseases – generally speaking – it is best to avoid all food containing sugar, even honey, and follow a low carb diet and the advice of a doctor you trust.

A specialist may administer certain honey varietals in large doses when treating some chronic diseases. There are success stories about healing cancer with huge amounts of honey, but for this you'll need the help and control of a knowledgeable specialist in this field or a special clinic.

Honey for stomach pain

As I described earlier, some honey varietals (in my case I used canola honey) may help with peptic ulcers, and with substantial dietary changes, along with a propolis tincture cure, I got rid of my ulcer completely (see *How I used Propolis against gastric ulcers*, page 115).

Stomach pains, of course, can be caused by other things, too. When they persist, it is best visit a doctor to determine the cause.

Honey for colds and influenza

Flu and colds are common illnesses with many uncomfortable symptoms: coughing, a runny nose, a sore throat, blocked sinuses, headaches, body aches, fever or chills. In fact when being infected I reduce the amount of honey I ingest a maximum of one-two tablespoons – 45-50 g – a day.

Honey for insomnia

Another experience I had with the beneficial effects of honey, changed my attitude towards it. It occurred that after a two days fasting I could not sleep well at night. I would fall asleep, but I woke up after 1-3 hours and couldn't get back to sleep. I had had some similar experiences before, but usually my sleeping pattern quickly returned to normal.

This time I was a zombie; I wasn't able to do my work properly during the day, nor was I able to sleep. Moreover, I had a serious fear of death, because I knew about the dangers of long-lasting insomnia.

I began taking high doses of melatonin when I would wake up after a few hours of sleep. Melatonin is normally produced by the pineal gland in our brain and it is a kind of sleep hormone. This helped me get a few more hours of sleep, but then I would wake up dizzy, which again made my work impossible.

Probably it wasn't an accident that I came across an article written about the beneficial properties of honey for insomnia. Actually, honey helps store glycogen in the liver, from where the brain will be fueled. The main sugar compounds of honey are easily metabolized and transformed into glycogen. If the glycogen stock is down in the liver, because of a bad diet during the day, the brain will suffer metabolic stress, as adrenalin and cortisol are released to solve the problem.

In my case, the signs of this metabolic stress might have been the higher heart rate I observed when I woke up after 1-3 hours of sleep in the night.

I started to eat two tablespoons of raw honey at bedtime.

Just after a few days I was sleeping about 4-5 hours in one stretch, which was much, much better than 1-3 hours. Also after being up for half an hour or so, I could get back to sleep for another 2-3 hours. In this second sleep I had very vivid dreams. The REM phase in which people have the most dreams is very important for establishing new neuronal structures in our brain. Ingesting honey at bedtime helped me develop better sleep patterns.

Actually, my insomnia wasn't solved completely, as some nights I couldn't get back to sleep, and 4-5 hours of sleep wasn't enough for the whole day.

Everyone has different needs, but it's acknowledged that the normal amount of sleep is seven to nine hours per night, or in a 24 hour period. Less than 6 hours of sleep results in 200% increased risk of having a heart attack or a stroke.

The body has a circadian rhythm – a kind of internal clock set by the cycle of light and dark. This circadian rhythm may be different in different individuals. You may be an early bird – a person who goes to bed early in the evening – , or you might be a night owl who prefers being up late at night and sleeps until late in the morning.

In our everyday life, we easily overlook this as, in many cases, our social life starts in the evening and most of us are living a night owl's life.

Unfortunately I am an early bird. No matter how late I go to sleep, I'm up often at about 4 a.m. In my earlier years I didn't really realize this, as falling back to sleep wasn't such an issue.

But a sleep specialist I visited had me acknowledge this and take it seriously. Beside this he advised me:

to keep a regular sleep routine, which means I have to go to bed (9.00 pm) and to wake up at the same time (5.30 a.m.);

to employ a pre-bed routine that signals that sleep is coming: I listen to classical music and read;

to prepare a cool, dark, and quiet environment for sleep;

to reduce caffeine and to avoid it completely after 12:00 pm.

to take a nap in the afternoon if I feel sleepy at 3-4 pm, but skip it after 4:30;

not to exercise 3-4 hours before bed- a short walk with the dog is okay;

to create a bedroom free of phones, tablets, computers;

to avoid blue light (screens) at least 3 hours before going to bed. They can disturb the circadian rhythm as they mimic daylight. I downloaded a blue-light reduction app for all my devices.

Though I cannot stick to all of these all the time, especially going to bed at 9.00 p.m., they help to improve my sleep patterns, just as honey does when I take it before bedtime, and I am resolved to get 7-7,5 hours sleep per 24 hours.

Sleep disorders can be caused by severe issues like sleep apnoea, bruxism etc. If your sleep disorder persists, it's advised to visit a sleep specialist as soon as possible.

Honey for obesity

According to some studies, honey helps control appetite and lose weight.[39] [40]

By consuming honey before bed (1 to 2 tablespoons), the body begins to burn fat during sleep.

Nonetheless, obesity can be a complex issue, so don't expect that eating honey will allow you to lose weight without making other lifestyle and dietary changes. Besides, obesity can be hormonally determined. There are also studies that link obesity to the changed gut microbiome.[41]

Anyway, taking one or two tablespoons of honey will probably help you lose some weight, given you take care of your diet as well.

I usually gain weight in the spring and at the beginning of summer, as I overeat when extracting honey. Then I have to be careful and when I want to lose some weight, I eat only 1 tablespoon of honey at bedtime.

Honey when consuming alcohol

Alcohol dehydrogenase is the enzyme that detoxifies alcohol in our liver, converting it to acetaldehyde and then to acetic acid. But the amount of cofactor, nicotinamide adenine dinucleotide (NAD), required for the enzyme's activity, is rapidly used up by these reactions.

> *When we eat honey, fructose helps our alcohol-stressed liver and the reduced NAD is renewed. Detoxification can go on.*

That's why it seems to be sensible to eat some honey before and after consuming alcohol in order to protect our liver and brain.[42]

Honey for massage

For our overall well-being, we need intimate moments. Massaging our partner or being massaged by her or him can be important parts of those moments.

> *Bees can also help with this, as honey, when added to oil, softens and hydrates our skin. Moreover, honey contains minerals, vitamin C and B6, folate and riboflavin and many more constituents, that's why its absorption into the skin appears to be beneficial.*

When using honey, the best massaging technique is to pull up your palms on the skin in a pumping motion. That'll stimulate the reflex zones and circulation.

A massage oil recipe with honey:

Mix five tablespoons of honey with 450-500 ml (two cups) of almond/olive/sesame oil and two tablespoons of rose oil (not essential oil). You can add a few drops of an essential oil of therapeutic value (lavender or lemon balm for relaxation, mint for refreshment etc.) as well.

Summary

- Honey can be immunostimulating and certain compounds of it are antimicrobial.

- Apalbumin 1, is a compound found in royal jelly and it is present in some honey types as well.

- Kynurenic acid (KYNA) – mainly present in chestnut honey.

- An enzyme called glucose oxidase in honey produces hydrogen peroxide, when there is free water available in the surroundings.

- The "healing" property of honey is due to its acidity as well, (the pH of honey is about 3.5).

- A compound called Methylglyoxal (MGO) is a powerful antibacterial agent present in Manuka honey from New Zealand. (Medihoney)

- Mild to mid-range injuries and second-degree burns seem to heal 4-5 days earlier when putting honey on them than with clinically used Silver sulfadiazine. (Chestnut honey in Vivamel, Manuka honey in Medihoney)

- Some honey varietals (canola, chestnut, manuka) may help with peptic ulcers. With substantial dietary changes, and along with a propolis tincture cure, some may get rid of ulcers for the long term as well.

- Stomach pains, can be caused by other pathogens, too. When they persist, it is best to visit a doctor to determine the cause.

- Flu and colds are common illnesses with many uncomfortable symptoms. When being infected it's best to reduce the amount of honey to a maximum of one tablespoon (22-28 g a day).

- If the glycogen stock is down in the liver, because of a bad diet during the day, the brain will suffer metabolic stress at night, as adrenalin and cortisol are released to solve the problem and we may wake up. One or two tablespoons of honey at bedtime may solve this, but insomnia can be a complex issue.

- Taking one or two tablespoons of honey at bedtime will probably help you lose some weight, if you take care of your diet as well.

- When using honey, the best massaging technique is to pull up your palms on the skin in a pumping motion.

8. HONEY RECIPES

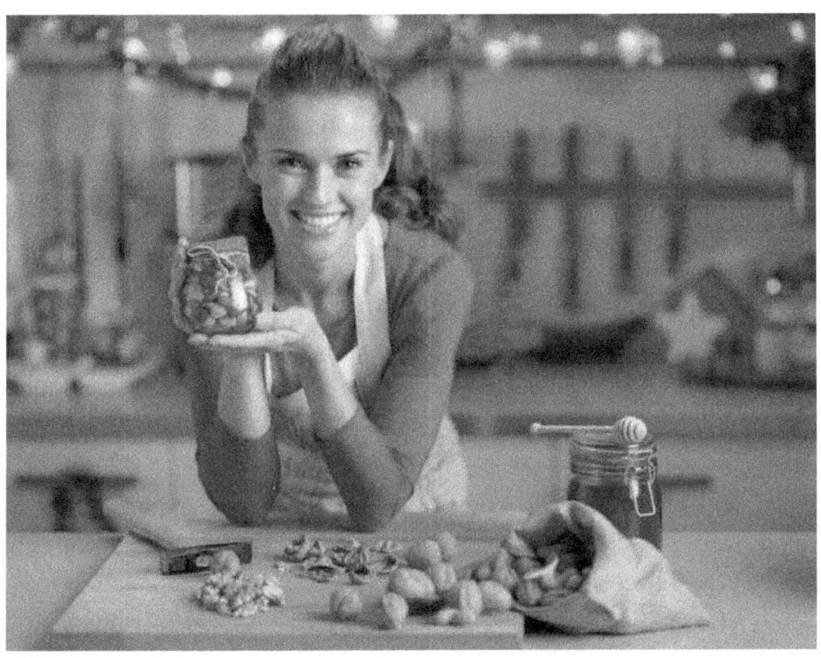

In this section you'll learn:

- Why and how to prepare simple honey recipes with walnuts, sesame seeds, yogurt etc.;

- How to infuse honey with fruits, herbs or spices;

- How you can make your own creamed honey;

- How to make a honey gingerbread men;

Every great thing is simple!

At least this statement applies to the recipes here.

> *Don't hesitate to try them. It won't take too much time to prepare these recipes and then enjoy the benefits of honey and the other healthy ingredients.*

Offering some to your guests will be also a great idea!

They are tasty and when consumed moderately are good for our health.

I also offer some of them to my customers at the market: Chocolate-Honey, Honey with Turmeric and Black Pepper, Honey with Walnut, Infused Honey.

I rarely use honey for baking as the important compounds in honey get destroyed by high temperature and only the carbohydrates and sugars will remain and then will probably be metabolized the same way as table sugar or HFCS would be. But of course, I sometimes eat gingerbread-men when my wife prepares some around Christmas. You'll find her recipe here as well.

Honey with walnuts

The best honey varietal for this recipe is one with a higher ratio of fructose to glucose, like acacia, chestnut, etc. All honey varietals that stay liquid for longer are suitable.

> *Walnuts are considered very healthy, as they contain protein, saturated fats, monounsaturated fats and polyunsaturated fats. They have lots of omega-3 and 9 fatty acids and ellagic acid which is a natural antioxidant.*

It is believed that walnuts help with high blood pressure, anemia and stomach ulcers. In ancient Rome they were used as aphrodisiacs. Therefore the combination of honey and walnuts is a healthy choice.

Ingredients:
For a mixture of 100-120 grams – for one/two portion(s)
- *2 tablespoons of liquid acacia/chestnut honey,*
- *2 tablespoons of walnuts;*

Method:
Mix equal parts honey and nuts. Serve in small cups.
You may also grind the walnuts if you prefer. I personally enjoy eating them in honey without being ground.

Honey with sesame seeds

Theoretically 3-4 tablespoons of sesame seeds can provide your calcium need per day (1000 mg). But it also contains copper and zinc. Roast the sesame seeds, then wait till they have cooled down. Then mix equal parts honey and sesame seeds together.

Honey-Chocolate

Chocolate, as usually manufactured, contains added sugar and soya lecithin. All this is not highly appreciated by reform nutritionists. But cocoa itself, one of the main constituents of chocolate bars, has unbelievable benefits for our health.

It is rich in polyphenols, which improves blood flow to our brain. It may lower the risk of stroke or reduce high blood pressure. It is beneficial to depression. It is immunostimulating, it may help with controlling obesity.

The recipe below makes chocolate a healthy choice you can prepare easily and quickly. Use high quality cocoa!

The advantage of canola honey (or any honey with a higher glucose ratio) for this recipe is that it crystallizes relatively quickly and it has a "creamy" rather than hard crystal consistency. That allows it to be used as a base for chocolates, or toppings. For therapeutic uses I prepare this recipe with acacia or chestnut honey.

The following recipe is for about 110-130 grams of "Honey-Chocolate". You may experiment with the ingredients, but the following ratio suits my taste best. My wife prefers it with less coconut oil.

Materials:

- *2 tablespoons of canola honey (you may also use other honey varietals with high glucose to fructose ratios, but in my region canola proved to be best for the base of this chocolate recipe.)*
- *1.5 tablespoon of coconut oil;*
- *1 tablespoon of high cocoa butter containing cocoa;*

Method:

Warm up the coconut oil, (don't let it be hot!) Add the cocoa and stir until it's homogenized.

Then add the honey and stir until it is mixed with the coconut oil and cocoa.

While letting it cool down stir it once or twice so that the whole mixture is more or less homogenized.

If hazelnuts or other nuts are added it is a real delicacy, and can satisfy cravings.

You can use it as a topping for cakes or as a dressing for the previous recipes with nuts and sesame seeds!

Cooling it down (the canola honey version) and leaving it in the fridge can result in a harder consistency and you can serve it as chocolate bars. Otherwise (the version with acacia honey/liquid honey), you may serve it in cups.

Honey with yogurt

It's a good idea to put honey in yogurt, one teaspoon per cup. I rarely eat milk products, except cheese. But sometimes I receive homemade goat's milk yogurt from a good friend of mine and I really enjoy it with acacia honey and walnuts. It seems to be very beneficial to the gut microbiome. My friend offers his yogurt with acacia honey as well at the local market and it is very popular. You can add some fruits, too.

Honey with fruits

Mix equal parts of honey and fruit. For one-two servings, you can take two tablespoons of honey and about 50-70 grams of fresh fruit. Liquid honey is the best for this. For fruits, you can use banana, strawberry, raspberry, blueberry, etc. This is a very good prebiotic, helping our microbiome.

Infused honey with herbs or spices

You may use one of the following: lavender, mint, cinnamon, anise, cardamom, vanilla. Of course, you may experiment with others too or mix them together. I really enjoy honey mixed with lavender or mint.

Ingredients:

- *1 kg acacia honey or a honey varietal with higher fructose content that stays liquid for longer;*

- *1-3 gram of dried herb/spice or 20-35 grams of fresh herbs (Honey will absorb the water and interestingly the herbs get dried in the honey!)*

Method:

Just pour honey on the herb in a jar and put it aside for a week, you may mix it and leave another few days. When mixing honey with ground spices (cinnamon, anise, cardamom etc.) stir or mix it regularly with a mixer.

Infusing honey with fruits and a lemonade

You have to be careful not to put too much fresh fruit into the honey, as it will raise the water content and spoil the honey and can cause yeast build up over time.

You can use refrigerated fruit, as well, after letting them warm up to room temperature. In 0.5 kg (1 pound) of honey add a maximum of 15-20 grams of fresh fruit, mix it and leave it for a few days.

Enjoy it as it is, without overeating! The flavor nuances that the honey gets from the fruit make the honey infused with fruit a perfect base for lemonades or homemade soft drinks.

Make a lemonade: mix one tablespoon of this infused honey with a glass (250-300ml) of water and some lemon juice.

Your own creamed honey:

As creamed honey can be expensive or you don't know how it's been produced – it could have been heated – you can make your own creamed honey.

A. If you have liquid honey, put it in the fridge for a few hours or one day until crystallization begins. That means it's no longer transparent, but has become opaque. This is the stage when you can still mix it with a strong mixer. Smaller mixers may not do the job.

   Some honey varietals with high fructose content can require more time to crystallize. Check it after a few hours in the fridge. Then take it out.

Mix the opaque honey with a mixer for a few minutes. The goal is to grind the crystals. The honey doesn't need to be put back into the fridge. Mix it each day for 3-5 minutes. Crystallization will result in finer crystals now. After a few days, when you can no longer mix it, as it would damage your mixer, just put it aside.

Making 2-3 kilos of honey at once in a large pot will allow you to use the mixer thoroughly.

B. If you have crystallized honey, you can decrystallize it first and just repeat the above steps. (See *Decrystallization*, page 77)

Lassi with honey

Lassi is a delicious Indian drink made from yogurt.
Ingredients for half a liter of Lassi:

- *150 ml (5 US fl. oz.) yogurt*

- *350 ml (12 US fl. oz.) water*

- *one or two tablespoons of honey*

Method:
Mix the ingredients then refrigerate.

Honey with turmeric and black pepper

The following recipe is great for preventing and fighting sore throats or beginning colds. You can easily prepare it on your own as well.

It is worth preparing half a kilo (one pound) of it, which you can keep in your home pharmacy for emergencies.

Keep in mind that even if you find it tasty (some find it awful) this is not for everyday consumption. When you need it for colds and flu, take it for only 2-3 days: Important: allow this "drug" to dissolve slowly in your mouth and don't drink or eat anything for half to one hour after taking it in order to let it work in your throat, mouth cavity and digestive system. Use it in preventive periods only for two to four days and don't take more than two to three half teaspoon of it a day.

Ingredients for a small amount – when preparing a larger amount just multiply the following:
- *100 grams honey (chestnut, lime, acacia, dandelion, buck-wheat from a local beekeeper);*
- *25 gram (a tablespoon) turmeric (powder);*
- *5 gram (a half to one teaspoonful) black pepper;*

Method:
Mix the ingredients thoroughly and let them rest for a while, then put it in small jars.

Honey-cheese spread

If you want to keep it simple, a spread can be prepared with honey and cream cheese by blending equal parts of honey and cheese together. But you may consider the following recipe as well, as it isn't too complicated:

Ingredients:
- *6-7 tablespoon (160gr – 5,6 oz) honey*
- *2-3 tablespoon (70 gr – 2,5 oz) cream cheese*
- *2 tablespoon (50-60 gr – 2 oz) coconut oil*
- *¼ teaspoon (4-6 gr – 0,2 oz) ground cinnamon (you may try it instead of cinnamon with cardamom as well.)*

Blend all the ingredients until the mixture is smooth. Spread it on crackers or toasts.

Honey- Gingerbread Men

Ingredients
Dough:

- 350 g (12.3 oz) all-purpose flour
- 1 teaspoon cinnamon
- ¼ teaspoon ginger
- ¼ teaspoon cloves
- 1 teaspoon baking soda
- 1 teaspoon vanilla extract
- 2 eggs
- 115 g (4 oz) butter
- 2 tablespoon honey (55-60 gr – 2oz) honey
- Glaze:
- 120g (4 oz) icing sugar
- 4 teaspoon milk
- food coloring

Method:
Mix flour with spices and baking soda. Add butter, eggs and honey, knead them into a dough, cover it and put it into the fridge for 1,5-2 hours.

Roll out the dough between two sheets of baking paper or on your lightly floured rolling board. You may use cookie cutters or a knife to cut your preferred gingerbread shapes.

Bake the dough for around 15 minutes in an oven preheated to 180°C (358°F), then let it cool completely.

While the dough is cooling you can mix the icing sugar with milk and food coloring. Using a slightly cut piping bag put it onto the cooled dough. You may write or draw with the glaze on the cake.

Summary

- Enjoy the benefits of honey and the other healthy ingredients in these easy recipes.

- Walnuts contain protein, saturated fats, monounsaturated fats and polyunsaturated fats, lots of omega 3 and 9 fatty acids and ellagic acid, which is a natural antioxidant. It is believed that walnuts help with high blood pressure, anemia and stomach ulcers.

- A few tablespoons of sesame seeds can provide your calcium need for the day, but they contain copper and zinc as well.

- Cocoa is rich in polyphenols improving blood flow to our brain. It may lower the risk of stroke or reduce high blood pressure. It is beneficial to depression. It is immunostimulating and may help with controlling obesity.

- Honey with (goat) yogurt seems to be very beneficial to the gut microbiome

- Mix equal parts of honey and fruits.

- Experiment infusing honey with lavender, mint, cinnamon, anise, cardamom, vanilla etc.

- Infuse honey with small amounts of fruits. Eat it or use it for lemonades.

- Make your own creamed honey by putting honey into the fridge then mixing it regularly with a mixer.

- Lassi is a delicious prebiotic drink made from yogurt

- Honey with turmeric and black pepper is great for preventing and fighting sore throats or beginning colds.

- Make a simple a spread by blending equal parts of honey and cheese together. You may also consider a more complex recipe as well.

9. PROPOLIS

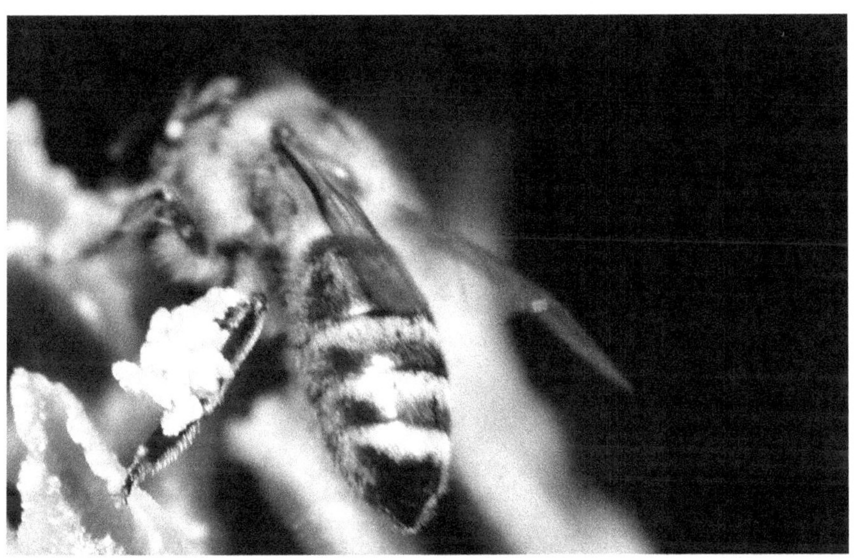

In this section you'll learn:

- What propolis is and where it comes from;

- How to use propolis for injuries, sores, different infections, gastric ulcers etc;

- How to prepare propolis tincture, honey with propolis;

- How to use propolis as a spice;

What is propolis?

Bees collect the resins of local trees/bushes just as they collect pollen. The bees use these resins to make propolis. They mix them with wax and use it to disinfect the hive or decrease the size of its entrance and to fill in the cracks.

When a "bigger" honey hunter (e.g. a mouse) gets into the hive, the bees kill it by stinging it to death and as they cannot easily carry out its corpse, they cover it with propolis so that it doesn't infect their environment.

There are scientific data that convincingly demonstrate that propolis has a direct regulatory effect on basic functional properties of immune cells.

> *Thus propolis can be considered as a powerful natural anti-inflammatory medicine influencing different types of immune-responses, probably via immunoregulatory T cells.*[43]

Caffeic acid phenethyl ester (CAPE) and chrysin are present in propolis extracts in different concentrations. They are responsible for the antioxidant, antimicrobial, anti-inflammatory and anticancer properties of propolis.[44]

Researchers have also identified artepillin C in Brazilian green propolis as having potential antitumor properties.

CAPE and artepilin C suppress cancer cell proliferation via their anti-inflammatory effects, decrease cancer stem cell populations, block specific oncogene signaling pathways, and modulate the tumor microenvironment.[45]

The issue with propolis is that its composition varies depending on the location of the bees and which plants they have access to.

Propolis from Central Europe won't have the same makeup as propolis from Brazilian bushes.

If you experience any negative effects stop taking or using it. If you aren't sure, talk to your doctor before taking propolis, especially if you have existing asthma or allergies.

If you would like to use it as an additional treatment for a chronic disease, discuss this with your doctor as well.

Using propolis as a preventive remedy, you can enjoy the advantages it provides your immune system.

How to use propolis for sores, injuries, cuts, skin rashes

You can use a propolis tincture for inflammation and sores inside the mouth (oral mucositis), canker sores (Aphthous stomatitis), or outside the mouth, like cold sores (Herpes simplex), or for injuries, burns, cuts or different skin breakouts by putting it on them. If needed you can use cotton wool.

For injuries, cuts, skin rashes and areas of skin irritation, severe dryness such as psoriasis or eczema it is very simple to apply it. Just put it on whatever you'd like to cure, then let it dry it and form a film.

If using the recipe I recommend here (it is a very thick one), it can smear onto things or your clothes, so you may use a bandage if you think it is necessary.

For sores inside your mouth, you can use cotton wool to put propolis on the spot you'd like to rub. If you can't reach the spot, put some propolis in your mouth and let it run over the spot.

Remember that using propolis may help and reduce symptoms, but its effect can be even better or longer lasting if you make some diet or lifestyle changes or improve your sleeping patterns.

Propolis for stomach pain

As you read at the beginning of this book, I got rid of my bilious spasms and most of my reflux with a dietary change – a low carb, gluten- and milk-free diet.

But I still had a sensitive stomach: some reflux and stomach pain after eating certain foods, like carbohydrates or honey (except canola honey). And sometimes I have woken up at night with a burning pain in my stomach and upper abdomen. This pain can signal a serious illness. It may be advisable to visit the doctor. In my case it turned out I have peptic ulcer.

Peptic ulcers are commonly caused by bacteria called Helicobacter pylori or in certain cases by non-steroidal anti-inflammatory drugs.

H. pylori was first identified as causing peptic ulcers in the late 20th century by Barry Marshall and Robin Warren, who received the Nobel Prize in Physiology and Medicine in 2005 for their discovery.

Since then it's been scientifically proven that propolis strongly inhibits Helicobacter pylori.[46]

How I used propolis against gastric ulcers

My first propolis cure for my stomach pain caused by a peptic ulcer looked like this:

I kept a two-day fast. This may seem drastic if you are not used to fasting, especially since propolis has an appetizing effect.

I mitigated the hunger by drinking some water or tea (without sugar or honey). However, I didn't drink (or later eat) right after I'd taken propolis. I waited at least one hour.

I drank 20-30 ml of water with 1 teaspoon (about 50-60 drops) of dense propolis three times the day (morning, noon, evening).

From the third day on, I started to eat a meal in the evening and a tablespoon of canola honey, while I continued with the propolis intake for 3 more days.

In my diet during this cure of one week I ate various well-cleaned fresh or boiled vegetables, boiled eggs, or thoroughly prepared meat and natural fats. I avoided carbohydrates like sugar, bread, cakes, chocolates etc. and fruits, milk/milk products, margarine.

After returning to my normal diet, I could eat all kinds of honey varietals without experiencing stomach pain. Of course I continued with my low carb diet.[i]

Nowadays I would do this the same way, only I would also take magnesium, probiotics, vitamin C, B-complex and D.

Sometimes I still get stomach or intestinal infections, but I can clearly feel and detect when this happens, and then I repeat what I did on the first two days of my cure just described.

It is important to know that if you use the above method against ulcers and your pain doesn't cease after a few days visit a doctor as soon as possible!

Why long-term use is not advised

While propolis isn't considered a high risk product, I know that some beekeepers who collected propolis without gloves have developed a kind of propolis allergy, an eczema-like outbreak.

I also know a middle-aged beekeeper colleague who took one or more grams of raw propolis each time he worked with his hives. He would take the propolis directly from the hive, chew it a bit then swallow it.

He thought this was a healthy preventive measure against pathogens. But one day, after many years of this practice, he felt an annoying discomfort and fell in bed depressed with no special symptoms. He went for clinical analyses, but the doctors couldn't easily diagnose the problem. Finally, an endoscopic analysis showed sediment in his intestinal tract.

---

[i] I mention my "low-carb" diet throughout this book, but probably my diet isn't a real low-carb diet, as I eat a good deal of honey, fruit and food containing resistant starch. Anyway, I keep away from added sugar and too much starch and cakes.

While this individual case is not scientific evidence, it is an indication that more research is needed in this respect.

You'll see if you try to make propolis infused oil that raw propolis doesn't dissolve easily.

I am sharing the story of this beekeeper because even if propolis isn't considered a high risk product, you must be careful and only take it for a shorter periods of time so your body can naturally get rid of the possible sediments.

Of course, propolis tincture works in a very different way than raw propolis does when it comes to sediments. We don't know that it would build sediments, but there is no scientific research on this topic and we can't be sure.

Apitherapy enthusiasts who read the first edition of this book were critical of my precautions with raw propolis and using it for short or moderate periods of time. I'm so sorry that I've disappointed them, but I think a healthy precaution is absolutely necessary in self-treatment, though perhaps someday science will prove that I wasn't right in this respect.

Warning

Propolis isn't recommended for those who are allergic to pollen. You should be also very careful when using it with small children or infants.

You may find recommendations to use propolis for some chronic diseases, as well as cancer, liver and kidney infections etc. While there may exist studies that confirm the potential of propolis for many chronic diseases, I don't advocate trying to heal these illnesses on your own. For all those cases, consult a trained expert in apitherapy.

Products with propolis

You may find ointments and lipsticks containing propolis, and probably other products will be developed as well as its benefits become more widely known. I recommend, along with other beekeepers and apitherapists, to use these products intermittently for the aforementioned reason – allergies can develop.

Where to purchase propolis for your home pharmacy and your kitchen

You can buy propolis tincture, ointments, or honey containing propolis from some pharmacies, shops or beekeepers in your local market. I think any of these sources are okay.

If you want to prepare your own propolis product, buy raw propolis from a local beekeeper, thus you can control the density and the consistency of it.

Propolis tincture

I think this is a must in every household! In most of the recipes and products in the pharmacies, you will find propolis tincture prepared in a 1/9 propolis/alcohol ratio. Many apitherapists advocate a 5% propolis tincture!

Preparing the following recipe will result in a dense tincture (1 part raw propolis, 2 parts alcohol).

You'll need:
- *A dark jar with a lid*
- *30 grams of raw propolis*
- *60 grams of clear grain (pure) 96 degree alcohol.*

Cut the propolis with a sharp knife or just tear it into small pieces, if you can. You can also try to grind it, but as the propolis can be waxy or hard (depending on how it has been stored or what source it comes from) grinding may not work and it may destroy your grinding machine!)

You can put these small pieces in the alcohol.

But if you want to have a denser tincture, put the small propolis pieces in your freezer overnight then grind it with a coffee grinder right after taking it out of the freezer.

Put the small pieces of propolis or the ground propolis in the alcohol in a dark jar, close the lid and store it in a dark place at room temperature for 2-4 weeks. Shake or stir (if you prepare a larger amount) it regularly each day. Then strain it with a cheesecloth or paper coffee filter.

The color of this tincture is brownish to dark black-brown. Store it in a dark bottle and dark place.

There is no evidence that it will lose its potency after years but if there is some left after 3-5 years, renew your stock.

This tincture is good for injuries, cuts, rashes, sores.

In preventive periods put half or a full teaspoon of this tincture in a small amount of water (20-30ml- 0,7-1 US fl. oz.) half an hour before your meals. Use it for 2-4 days!

Advice for beekeepers preparing propolis tincture

If you are preparing a few liters of the tincture for your customers, shaking and straining and packaging could be a messy act. For this reason, use a larger jar with a large opening so that you can easily stir (not shake!) it each day. After 2-4 weeks don't strain it but stop stirring it. Let it settle overnight. With an appropriate syringe, you can now measure it into small bottles.

What if you don't use alcohol, even in small amounts

You may let the alcohol evaporate from the tincture by warming it in a double-boiler. An oily sediment will remain. You can add this to olive oil or fat and stir it thoroughly. Or the other way to avoid alcohol is that you prepare Propolis Infused Oil (see below)

Propolis Infused Oil

Before preparing it keep in mind that Propolis Infused Oil can be time and patience consuming to make as it needs temperature control, then a long stirring period.

Use pots that you won't use anymore for other things. Be sure the propolis you are using is not too waxy.

Ingredients:
- *10 grams raw propolis (about 1-2 TBS)*
- *200 ml (7 oz) olive oil (other oils or fats can be used as well)*

Method:
Use a double boiler and a thermometer to control the temperature. Don't heat it over 50°C (122°F) as high temperatures may destroy the beneficial compounds in the propolis. Stir and heat the materials for at least 30 minutes and up to 2-4 hours. Not all of the propolis will dissolve.

Strain this mixture through a cheesecloth or a paper coffee filter. You may have to filter the oil twice. Store it in a sealed jar in a dark place.

Propolis as a spice

Propolis tincture, if dense enough can give a very special flavor to different foods. Especially sweet creams for cakes get a rich, intense flavor from it. A few drops or a teaspoon will do.

Honey with propolis

A dense mixture:
Add 50 ml (1,7 US fl. oz.) propolis tincture in 200 gram honey and stir it while warming up the honey to about 35-40°C (95-104°F). Be sure not to overheat it.

Honey Propolis Throat Spray

Put the undiluted propolis tincture in a spray bottle.
Or mix three tablespoons of propolis tincture with two tablespoons of honey and one tablespoon of warm water. Put it in a spray bottle. If you have the time to experiment, you can also mix different other herbal tinctures into it as well (echinacea, ginger etc.).

Summary

- Bees collect the resins of local trees/bushes just as they collect pollen.

- Caffeic acid phenethyl ester (CAPE) and chrysin are present in propolis extracts in different concentrations. They are responsible for the antioxidant, antimicrobial, anti-inflammatory and anticancer properties of propolis.

- For injuries, cuts, skin rashes and areas of skin irritation, severe dryness such as psoriasis or eczema it is very simple to apply.

- Propolis inhibits Helicobacter pylori.

- Long-term use of propolis is not advised.

- Don't chew or eat raw propolis, your gastric acid won't be able to dissolve it.

- Propolis isn't recommended for those who are allergic to pollen. Be also very careful when using it with small children or infants.

- Ointments, lipsticks and other products containing propolis should be used intermittently.

- You can buy propolis tincture, ointments, honey containing propolis and honey propolis throat spray, or prepare them yourself.

10. BEE VENOM

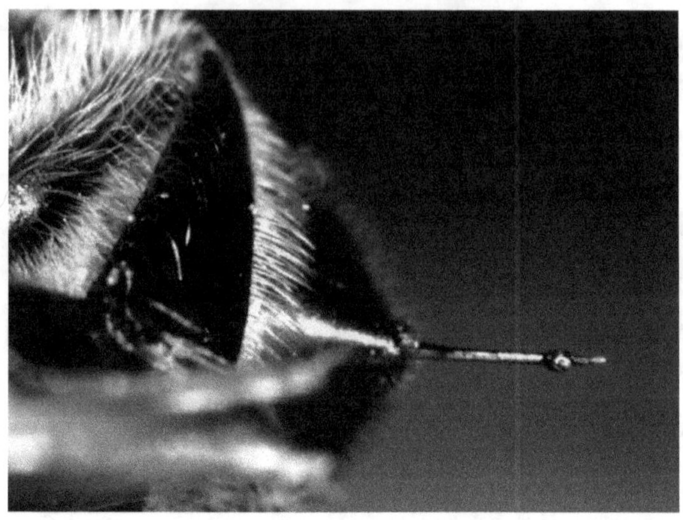

In this section you'll learn:

- How to use bee stings in practice;

- A massage with bee venom cream;

- The compounds of bee venom and how bee venom works;

- How to desensitize a hyper-allergy to bee venom

- Risks and lethal doses;

- History of bee venom therapy;

- Some success stories, an innovation and a proposal by a specialist for a Covid-protocol.

Another terrible flu experience of mine

As I mentioned before, for some unknown reason, I used to be susceptible to different infectious diseases. In the last 15-16 years – probably thanks to some lifestyle changes – I handle the flu, colds or stomach/intestinal pains that I catch once or twice a year relatively easily.

But a few years ago, after flying home from the Middle East, I fell ill for two weeks with a flu-like condition.

Usually I can prevent infection at the very beginning when the first signs appear. This time, as I was abroad, I couldn't carry out my usual preventive measures like fasting for a few days, taking propolis and honey, gargling with baking soda etc. In retrospect, the basic mistake was that I had no propolis tincture.

Since my first longer lasting flu-experience I hadn't been to the doctor to get rid of colds for about 30 years. This time I also wanted to heal without external help.

But unfortunately, my illness worsened in the third week and I started to cough constantly in a very annoying way. The cough ceased only for a little while during the day and it was very bad at night.

My wife was determined to call the doctor, not only because she was worried about me, but also because she and my son couldn't sleep well during the night due to my loud coughing.

I had to admit that this time my flu was different and I couldn't wait for my usual and rapid self-healing process. And after all I could not make my family suffer for my stubbornness in not wanting to see a doctor.

But I didn't want to give up easily, so I asked my wife for more patience and her help.

I thought that this could be a good opportunity to try out bee sting therapy on myself.

My wife unwillingly drove me to my hives. I took out a frame with bees from one of my best colonies (by the way it isn't a good idea for the bees to be removed or disturbed in the winter time) and put it quickly into my demonstration glass hive that I use for educational purposes. And we drove home.

I was not new to the subject of bee venom therapy. I had studied it for a while before writing some articles about it.

With my constant cough, I tried to refresh my knowledge and I re-read the available literature.

Studies report that besides its anti-inflammatory properties, bee venom possesses anti-mutagenic[47], anti-nociceptive (blocking the detection of pain)[48], radioprotective[49] (protecting against damage caused by microwaves) and anti-cancer effects.[50]

One study states its toxicity still prevents its use as an anti-inflammatory agent. But melittin could possibly be used for anti-inflammatory purposes if careful provisions are taken and technical developments help to transform it into a safe therapeutic agent.[51]

The good news is that there is such "a technical development" (See in chapter *A promising innovation*, page 150)

Bee venom has been used in treating rheumatoid arthritis, amyotrophic lateral sclerosis, Parkinson's disease, Alzheimer's disease, liver fibrosis, atherosclerosis, Lyme diseases, cancer to name just a few.

> *Like other bee products, bee venom works multifactorially: it has a regulating effect on our immune system and its compounds inhibit or destroy pathogens, i.e. its toxin – melittin – can poke holes in the protective envelope surrounding viruses.*

Bee venom has recently been used in many antiaging cosmetics against wrinkles.

When considering bee venom therapy – this applies to allopathic or other therapies as well – one has to weigh the risks, the gravity of his or her recent condition and the benefits of such a therapy.

Identifying acupuncture points – Bees in the jar

After refreshing my knowledge of the subject, I identified the Chinese acupuncture points on my body for cold. lung and improving immunity. As one of the most accessible acupuncture points of the lung (LU7) is very close to a vein I decided to apply the stings on the outside part of my wrist. Then I made a plan.

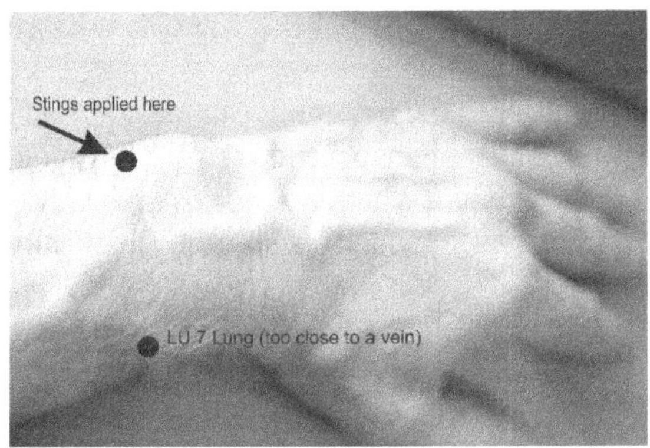

I put some honey in a jar and pressed its opening to the entrance of the observation hive. Some bees entered the jar then I closed the jar with a perforated lid.

Before applying the stings I put the jar of bees in the fridge for a few minutes so that I could handle the slowed down bees more easily, otherwise they would fly away when trying to catch them with the forceps. Care is needed not to leave the bees in the fridge too long as they can enter a state of torpor and won't be willing to sting.

As I am a chronic disease free person, the first step before applying bee sting therapy is that one must know whether she or he is allergic to bee venom.

Though I'm a beekeeper and I am exposed regularly to bee stings and I know that I am not hyper allergic to bee venom I've learnt on my own account that this may change from one moment to other (see in *Getting an anaphylactic shock and desensitization*, *page 136*).

The first sting was to determine whether I'd become allergic to bee stings or not. That means it is a diagnosis about my immune system.

It actually shows whether it is overreacting or underreacting to pathogens.

I took out a bee with the tweezers and applied the first sting one inch above my left wrist.

It showed no swelling or redness and I didn't experience accelerated heart beats or any nettle-rash on my body, even after 15-20 minutes. These would have been the symptoms of a hyper-allergy.

It was clear I was not allergic to bee venom, but it was also obvious that my immune system was not reacting well.

Then I applied the next stings until the first mild reaction come and the stung spot started to swell. This only happened after the 8th sting.

My coughing stopped in the evening which was almost unbelievable to me and which left my wife astonished, as she had skeptically watched my actions.

I still didn't feel well and I had to stay in bed, but I was overcome with relief. The next day I repeated my sting therapy on my right wrist adding an additional sting to the amount of the previous day – that meant 9.

In the evening I felt better and the next day I was able to do office work at my computer in my study. It took me all in all six days of therapy to totally recover and go back to work at the school where I was teaching.

During the six days of therapy, each day I added an additional sting to the previous ones. On the last day there were 13 stings.

I tried out different acupuncture points. Some were less and others were more painful spots on the body. The points above the wrists seemed to be the best for me.

After the therapy, the spots where I applied the stings the most were full of lesions. I cured them using the propolis tincture.

What apitherapist do differently

Trained experts in apitherapy carry out fewer sessions a week and apply stings to different parts of the body on a rotating basis, so the lesions caused by stings may heal better.

> *To reduce the initial pain of the sting, an ice-pack from the freezer can be applied for a few minutes to numb the sting site.*

Apitherapists apply a test sting before applying full stings to be sure that the patients aren't hyper-allergic. After letting the bee sting their patient they scratch out the stinger within a second. Then they wait for 15-20 minutes. If symptoms associated with anaphylaxis, such as loss of blood pressure, fainting, and breaking out in hives all over the body appear, the therapy must be stopped.

An epinephrine (adrenaline) injector and a kit must be on hand! Epinephrine is a medication used to treat a number of conditions, including anaphylaxis that can be caused by bee venom.

Bee venom acts on local and distant areas

Local areas are those where someone complains of symptoms. Distant points are points distant from the area of main complaint.

The latter are those which for some reason of reflex action or physiology relate to the area of complaint. Acupuncture points are found to be effective points where bee stings should be applied.[52]

That is probably one of the reasons why, in my case, the bee stings helped stop my coughing attack on the first evening.

Finding the spot to apply bee stings

Charles Mraz's[*] technique for choosing a sting site was looking for "hot spots" by pressing along the joints and bones. He called hot spots

---

[*] Charles Mraz is another person who did a lot for modern Bee Venom Therapy. He initiated clinical research in different institutes in the US and developed the USDA purity standard for dried whole venom and supplied venom to pharmaceutical companies internationally.

those parts of the body which are sensitive and aching when being firmly pressed. When found, he had marked them with a pen or marker.

It is interesting that these "hot spots" often coincide with the places where acupuncturists insert their needles. Using these points in bee sting therapy gives better results than other areas.[53]

Heavily inflamed areas or sites of the body not yet recovered from previous treatment shouldn't be stung.

A meridian massage with bee venom cream

After my first adventurous and successful therapy with bee stings, I attended Dr. Stefan Stangaciu's apitherapy course (available also online, see apitherapy.com) and learnt, amongst many other interesting techniques, a spine massage with bee venom cream.

When I feel the need, which means I feel that I am coming down with some infection, I let my wife give me this massage and also let her apply some bee stings on my spine and the neighboring meridians.

> *This massage is also effective without bee stings and is as follows:*

I. Application of the bee venom cream:

Apply bee venom cream in a line on the spine (1, 2 – see picture) starting from the first vertebra until you reach the last palpable vertebra on the neck.

Then measure the width of two thumbs (of the patient) to the right and the same to the left from the spine (line 1) and apply the bee venom cream downwards in lines parallel to the spine.

Now strike the spine with the lower part of your thumb pressed by the other thumb from the basic vertebra upwards (1,2).

Now measure the width of four thumbs (of the patient) to the right and the same to the left from the spine (line 2) and apply the bee venom cream downwards parallel to the spine.

You have applied the cream now to five meridians. Massage by letting your thumbs strike the spine and the meridians in the form of an artesian fountain. This means, start from the base (the lowest vertebra on the spine) till the last palpable vertebra at the neck, then come down on the two next 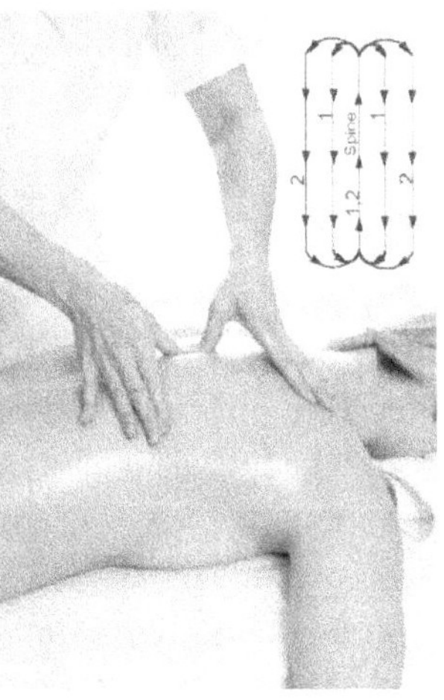 meridians, then back on the spine pressing it with both thumbs and coming down on the outer two meridians. Do this massage for about 3-5 minutes.

II. Finding the issues:

Now start pressing the spine meridian (1, 2) from the lowest vertebra cm by cm (inch by inch) going upwards. Stop where you find a sensitive point and stimulate that point by pressing for some time (3-5 minutes) with extra bee venom cream. (My wife marks a circle on this point with a marker to apply bee stings there later.)

Do the same downwards on each of the other meridians.

You may apply bee stings now on the points which you found problematic. First, be sure you are not hyperallergic to bee stings.

I usually sting myself with one sting at each problematic point. In my case my wife usually finds 3-4 such points when doing this massage.

If there is no swelling after the stings, I consider getting one more round of stings as the immune system needs some stimulus.

The practice of applying bee stings

If someone tries to apply bee stings, he or she will face some practical issues: How to take bees out of the hive? How to catch them with the tweezers?

There are different kits on the internet for this. However practical they may seem, their use needs lots of practice and mostly they are quite expensive. My kit, which I made for myself, is a very practical and inexpensive one.

As you see in the picture, it consists of simple surgical tweezers, a box for the bees and washers.

The box for the bees:

The wooden box has a sliding plexiglass lid with some small holes in it.

The big hole on the side serves to let some bees enter from the hive or from the jar. If you use a beehive entrance reducer and you attach the box to it, the bees will enter directly into the box.

Of course, this only works in the beekeeping season.

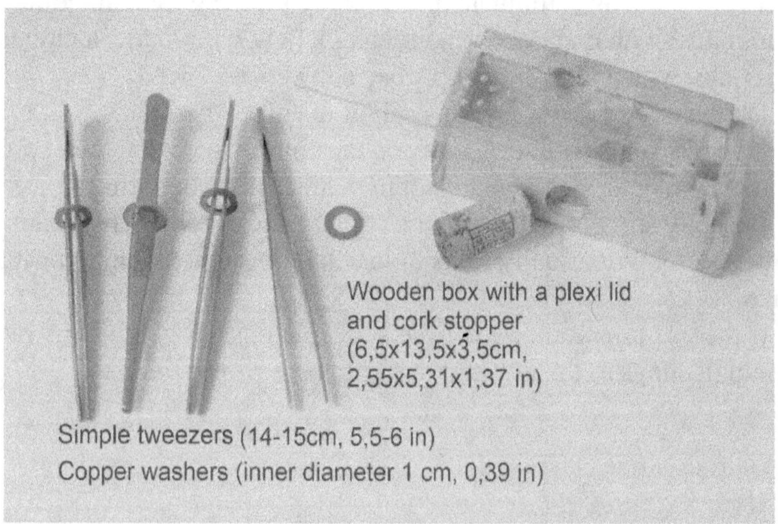

In the winter, if I need bees, I very gently brush some directly from the winter cluster into a jar, and then let them enter the box. If the winter cluster can't be seen on the top of the frames, I take out the last frame with bees and put it into my observation hive and let them enter the box from the observation hive. Such operations should be carried out very carefully as disturbing or destroying the winter cluster can be deadly for the whole colony.

The tweezers are simple surgical tweezers, they can be used with washers so that when you catch the bees from the box you can pull the washer down on the arm of the tweezers and the bee will stay caught till the sting is applied.

The box can be used for luring bees, as well. You can put some honey or sugar syrup into it, then open the lid halfway and put it outside. Bees, if there are some colonies in the area and they don't find mass blooming of some nectar-giving plant, will come around and sip from the syrup. Some wasps or flies may be also lured to the box, that is why I don't usually lure bees into the box in this way.

How to catch bees from the box

However simple it may seem, it isn't. The box I use has a sliding lid and a reduced entrance where the bees may come out when the lid is pulled a bit aside. But before you catch the bees they may quickly slip out from the box. So, it is best to put the box into the fridge (not into the freezer!) for a few minutes.

IMPORTANT: use an alarm clock or app, as forgetting about them and leaving them longer time in the fridge may kill them.

Take them out when they are slowed down but not completely hibernating. It's hard to say how many minutes you'll need, as different fridges may vary in temperature. Experiment with your fridge. I usually put the bees in the fridge for 5 minutes. Then if they haven't yet slowed down, I put them back for another 2-3 minutes. If they are still very active I repeat this as many times as necessary. (Set the alarm clock each time and don't kill the bees!)

How Does Bee Venom Work?

In my case, the bee venom therapy may have stimulated my immune system, which was obviously down, and awakened my body's reaction against pathogens.

When the stinger starts pumping venom into the body, large amounts of blood will flow to the stung site. The healing properties within the blood will concentrate around it.

The stingers should be left in the skin for at least 15-20 minutes so that all possible contents get into the body.

Adrenal glands stimulated by the venom release cortisol.[54] Cortisol is the natural version of cortisone, a steroid that is commonly used by physicians to treat chronic inflammation.

Note that cortisone is chemically not exactly the same as naturally produced cortisol. Cortisone treatment has its side effects and over a longer period, one can develop liver toxicity from it.

It's hypothesized that various B vitamins and vitamin C are needed for the body to produce cortisol.

For this reason, while applying bee stings I also took an extra dose of vitamin C and B multi-vitamins (about 2,000 milligrams of vitamin C – about a teaspoon of ascorbic acid powder and two pills of multi-vitamin B one hour before applying the stings.)

Another way bee venom probably helped me in this aggravated flu-like disease was due to the anti-inflammatory activity of its main component, melittin.[55]

Inflammation is actually a protective process of the body, however chronic inflammation can cause diseases like diabetes cardiovascular disease, rheumatoid arthritis, obesity, liver inflammation, asthma, inflammatory bowel disease, Amyotrophic Lateral Sclerosis and Parkinson's disease.

The compounds of bee venom

The compounds of bee venom are a tiny 26-amino-acid peptide called melittin, apamine, phospholipase A2,, mast cell degranulating peptide, adolapin, histamine, phospholipids, oligopeptides, saccharides, acid phosphatase and hyaluconidase, etc.[56]

Melittin is the principal constituent of this toxin (it constitutes about 50% of the weight of dried bee venom) and it works synergetically with phospholipase A2.

Normal "side effects" during a course of a therapy

The most common side effects are: initial pain of the sting, then swelling, redness, itching, soreness and tenderness, feelings of heat in the treatment area, and in extreme cases nausea and fever. None of these reactions are life threatening or mean that you've become hyper-allergic.

Reactive phase – the shift

If you didn't have side effects at the beginning of the therapy, the appearance of some is to be expected. It signals an immunological improvement and that a significant shift has taken place. Doctor Beck calls this the reactive phase and writes in his book that it is important to navigate the patients through this reactive phase: when one wants to get better he or she must stand the course.

Some may label this phase as an allergic reaction, which is not the case. It's important to realize the difference between these normal effects and hyper-allergy. In the second case it is imperative that one must stop with the bee venom therapy.

No effects of bee venom: a sign that it will work

In my case the first stings didn't cause any reaction. That signaled not only a weakened immune system but also that a bee venom therapy will work well for me.

Paradoxically that's the case in some other kinds of therapies. For example, when taking an extremely high dose of vitamin C, one should react with diarrhea. If this is not the case, that means that the therapy will work well for the patient. And when diarrhea comes that means the healing processes have started.

It is very similar with bee venom, when eventually symptoms come after being stung it means we are in the reactive phase.

Alcohol and antihistamines

No alcohol, in any form, should be used during the bee venom therapy, be it oral or applied at the sting site in order to disinfect it before being stung. This will negate the therapy.

As a beekeeper I learnt from my personal experience that I can develop a hyper-allergy at any time. That's why I keep a small amount of alcohol in the tool box I use when handling my hives. The best is to have an epinephrine (adrenaline) injector on hand as well. Actually when applying bee stings therapy a kit containing epinephrine is a must!

Antihistamines are used by many people against the uncomfortable reactions when being stung by insects.

When receiving bee venom therapy antihistamines are contraindicated as they suppress the immune system. We have to understand that the goal of bee venom therapy is to stimulate the immune system.

Hyper-allergy to bee venom

About one to two percent of the population is hyper-allergic to bee venom. It is also possible that someone becomes hyper-allergic to bee venom on the go, just as some beekeepers do (see below). If the person has not been stung within the past two to three weeks a test sting is always advisable.

As mentioned earlier, having an epinephrine injector on hand when applying bee venom therapy is a must.

Desensitization immunotherapy

If someone is hyper-allergic to bee venom, but for some reason he or she wants to get bee venom therapy or wants to become a bee-keeper, there is Venom Immunotherapy (VIT) available which involves a series of injections of increasing doses of bee venom over a period of years. It is very safe and efficient.

Getting an anaphylactic shock and desensitization

As I mentioned before I'd been around bees and hives since my childhood. But at a certain point in my late twenties I was overcome by shocking symptoms after being stung by a honey bee.

I wasn't handling our hives, I was just walking in our orchard when all this happened. I felt nauseous and had an accelerated heart rate. I had to lay down in the grass. Then a nettle rash developed on my arms and thighs. It was obvious to me that this was a hyper-allergic reaction to the bee venom.

I got frightened as I felt my nausea worsen and my heart beat even more quickly. After 20 minutes or so, these symptoms passed.

Luckily I recovered, but such a situation can even be deadly.

It is advisable for beekeepers to have some alcohol around when handling the bees to mitigate the overreaction of the body when such situations occur. It some cases it is best to have an epinephrine (adrenaline) injection on hand.

> *They used to use calcium, but that is no longer advised for bee venom hyper-allergic reaction. However calcium may have an important role when using bee venom.*[57]

In my experience, our bodies need more calcium when using bee venom. When I'm being stung by more than 5-6 bees while handling my hives or making a bee sting cure I feel slightly uncomfortable, which is normal as my body tries to counteract the effect of the venom. When I take some calcium, this feeling is barely noticeable. Some studies also suggest that calcium may play a role in the healing process when using bee venom. That's why I take it when being stung by bees. It also good to know that

> *the absorption and integration of calcium in our bodies is helped by active vitamin D, which we can get from at least 15 minutes in the sunshine each day.*

It is not clear why hyper-allergies develop in people already used to bee venom. It might be that the sting hits a vein or the venom contains an unusually high dosage of toxins.

Anyway, I had to avoid the hives unless I wanted to run the dangerous risk of anaphylaxis. The bees were not left alone, as my father handled them.

Not being able to go to my bees was a depressing perspective for me as I had always loved bees. Watching them and smelling the rich air of the hive were the most uplifting moments of my life, which is only comparable to some rare "breathtaking" life experiences.

Unfortunately, desensitization immunotherapy wasn't available at that time in my country. But later I told my story to someone who had just been cured out of a pollen allergy by a homeopath and he became personally involved in homeopathy.

He advised me to take high potentials of Apis mellifica globuli.

I have to admit that I am not too keen on homeopathy. In spite of being a bit skeptical, for a month I took 3x5 globuli a day of a middle range Apis available in the local pharmacy.

Then I took a bee allergy test at the clinic which came back negative. I nearly jumped out of my skin. I was able to approach the hives again.

When thinking about it now, I wonder whether the test would have been negative if I had taken it a few days after my hyper-sensitive reaction. It may had been a single bad situation, when the amount of melittin and some different unknown circumstances were in a favorable constellation for the overreaction.

I only became aware of the possibility of such a clinical test after I had completed the homeopathic Apis therapy.

Anyway I was happy to go back to see my bees.

Bee venom against a large range of diseases?

Bee venom can be an effective additive therapy for multiple sclerosis, Lyme disease, Parkinson's disease, cancer and Lou-Gehrig's disease as it diminishes neuroinflammation, inhibits programmed cell death of dopaminergic neurons, reestablishes normal dopamine levels, and safeguards against glutamate-induced neurotoxicity.

For the treatment of these conditions it is advisable to contact an apitherapist or a physician with expertise in apitherapy.

Bee venom can be also administered by injection or topically as a cream.

Is bee venom therapy dangerous?

Though there are lots of success stories about the effectiveness of bee venom therapy in treating different diseases, there are, at least at the moment, two reports about the dangerous or fatal outcomes of such therapy.

Currently we have to rely on anecdotal data which means that even though there are thousands of success stories and only a few stories relating the lethal or unfortunate outcomes of bee venom therapy, we do not know in statistical and scientific terms how bee venom therapies work in larger groups and control groups.

But as there are many ongoing treatments and some developers and researchers trying to capitalize on melittin, we'll probably have more statistical and clinical data in the near future.

When investigating the two unfortunate stories of bee venom application circulating on the internet, it turns out that in both cases the applier of bee stings/venom wasn't precautious enough, and, moreover, broke the rule for applying bee venom.

> *It is important to keep in mind when applying bee venom, besides being trained or knowledgeable in this area, one must have a kit containing an adrenaline injection (epinephrine) and he or she should know how to use it.*

Moreover, she or he should be familiar with different first aid treatments (laryngectomy, resuscitation etc.)

As it is instructive, let's take a closer look at these two cases.

The first case was reported in the Journal of Investigational Allergology and Clinical Immunology in 2018, by physicians of the Allergy Division, Ramon y Cajal University Hospital, Madrid, Spain.[58]

A 55-year-old Spanish woman decided to receive apitherapy at a private clinic to improve muscular contraction and stress. She had been attending bee sting therapy sessions every 4 weeks for 2 years when suddenly she developed a hypersensitive reaction. Right after a bee sting she had shortness of breath and sudden loss of consciousness.

The clinical personnel administered steroid medication (methylprednisolone), as unfortunately no adrenaline was available.

They called an ambulance which arrived 30 minutes later. Then a double dose of adrenaline (1 mg all in all), intravenous corticosteroids, saline infusion, and antihistamines were administered.

Upon arrival at the hospital the patient was intubated. A tomography scan indicated a watershed stroke, but the basic blood and the EKG results and chest x-ray were in the normal ranges.

The woman was hospitalized and in a coma, then died weeks later of multiorgan failure. This is the first reported case of someone who was tolerant to bee stings but during the treatment developed a hypersensitivity.

It's hard to say what would have happened if the personnel at the private clinic had administered an adrenaline injection right after the hypersensitive reaction.

Considering the fact that there are a century of records – since Dr. Phillip Terc or Dr. Bodog F. Beck accurately reported on their therapies – and we know of many other cases without lethal outcomes, probably the case of the 55-years-old Spanish woman would have had a better outcome if more precautions had been taken.

The second case you'll find circulating on the internet is the story of Gerard Butler's "adventure" with bee stings. He tells it on Late Night with Seth Meyers. He was advised by his nutritionist to try bee sting therapy for muscle strain that developed when working on his movie Geostorm. "I had heard of this guy injecting bee venom, because apparently it has many anti-inflammatory compounds."

The result of his bee venom "therapies": he was hospitalized twice.

It's worth watching the video and drawing some conclusions from it – watch on youtube: keywords: butler bee stings seth meyers. It actually relates a foolish therapy.

It's obvious that the "guy" who administered the bee venom to Butler wasn't aware of the basics and didn't stick to any known protocol.

Gerard Butler clearly relates this when telling that after he entered anaphylactic shock, the "naturopath", instead of applying an epinephrine injection or calling the ambulance, phoned his "instructor" to discuss the case.

We don't exactly know why he didn't apply epinephrine, there are some contraindications for it, but not calling immediately an ambulance was a real mistake. At least that's the conclusion based on the story related by Butler in this TV program.

But some other questions arise as well: Is it normal to want a rapid effect from a remedy for symptoms which could probably be solved with exercise, habitual changes, or even allopathic medicine? Of course people want instant healing for the issues they have because they just want to go on with their work or live their usual life.

One of the tasks for naturopaths and apitherapists is to help their patients understand that therapy is only part of the solution, they must make some lifestyle choices as well. The discovery of the causes is also important. The naturopath is just a knowledgeable helper in this process.

Another question arises in respect to Butler's story: How sensible is to go for treatment a second time when he has already experienced anaphylactic shock, which is a very serious thing, and he was obviously hypersensitive to bee venom? And why didn't anybody try to talk him out of it or advise him to desensitize first?

Yes, people are sometimes "maniacs" as Butler labels himself for his second trial of bee venom. Therefore double precaution is needed, both in making the decision to get bee venom therapy and in applying it.

When considering bee venom therapy – this applies to allopathic or other therapies as well – one has to weigh the risks, the gravity of his or her recent condition and the benefits of such a therapy.

The risks should in no way exceed the supposed benefits.

If someone is tortured by a really bad condition – see Ellie Lobel's case in the *Success Stories* – bee venom therapy can be a real consideration. But even in such cases, pondering and weighing the risks vs. the benefits is important and is the decision of the patient.

Risks, lethal dose and accidents

Bee venom, when used with precaution, seems to be safe for human treatments. The average lethal dose for an adult is 2.8 mg of venom per kg of body weight. In other words, a 75 kg person has a 50% chance of surviving injections of 210 mg of bee venom.

If each bee injects all its venom at a maximum of 0.3 mg venom per sting, 700 stings could well be fatal for such a person. For a child weighing 12 kg, as little as 112 stings could be deadly.

But most human deaths result from one or a few bee stings due to sensitive reactions, heart failure or choking from swelling around the neck or in the mouth.

Some history of bee sting therapy

Bee and wasp venom therapy was practiced in ancient Egypt, but we don't really know much about that. Hippocrates used it to treat arthritis and joint pain. It's claimed that the emperor Charlemagne regularly received bee venom treatment.

Bee sting therapy in modern Europe began with Dr. Philip Terc, who is regarded as the father of apitherapy.

Dr. Terc, who was a general practitioner in Marburg suffered from rheumatism (in Austrian Styria- now Maribor, Slovenia). One day in 1864 he was attacked and stung by a group of honey bees. To his surprise, from then on his rheumatic pains began to vanish and his limbs regained more flexibility.

Fascinated by this experience, he thought that the clinical studies by Dr. Lukomsky in Russia, regarding the beneficial effects of bee stings, should be taken seriously.

He only started experimenting with bee stings 11 years after his accident. His first patient for bee stings was a woman who had been treated by many physicians before, even by Terc, for deafness and cranial neuralgia without any improvement.

The physician, remembering his experience with the bees, started to apply bee stings to her on a daily base. Sometimes up to 90!

Though there was no improvement at first in her condition, fortunately the stings didn't have any negative effect either on his patient.

One day Terc applied 15 stings on her shoulders and neck and the woman was cured from her condition.

Terc went on with his research and experiments for the next ten years with outstanding results.

In 1888, in his "Report on the Peculiar Connection between Bee Stings and Rheumatism", we can read about his treatment of 660 patients with rheumatic arthritis to whom he applied almost 40 000 bee stings. The results: 82 % of them had a perfect cure- 544 patients; 15% had some improvement – 99 patients; and 3% experienced no relief – 17 patients.

Terc was convinced by these results that almost all true arthritis and rheumatism can be completely and lastingly cured with bee stings, except the cases in which the joints already have been damaged and ossification has taken place.

After hard and uninterrupted labor he decided to present his results about thousands of patients effectively cured at the University of Vienna.

Instead of being welcomed, he met a hostile and narrow-minded audience. Terc left Vienna fearing that he'd be interned in an insane asylum just as Ignaz Philipp Semmelweis had been less than 20 years before. His lecture remained unpublished by the University.

Misunderstood and ridiculed by the ruling medical authorities, he followed the fate of trailblazers such as Franz Anton Mesmer, Louis Pasteur, Philipp Semmelweis, and many others.

Later a Hungarian émigré physician, Bodog F. Beck, was the first to describe bee venom therapy in detail at the beginning of the 20th century in the US. He made a good career in New York applying bee venom for conditions that seemed beyond healing. His book *The Bible of Bee Venom Therapy* is one of the basic and most systematic books on the subject. Dr. Beck had good therapeutic results using apitherapy for muscular rheumatism, acute rheumatic fever, myositis, myalgia, neuritis, neuralgia, migraine, endocarditis, acute chronic arthritis, chronic surgical inflammation of the soft and bony tissues, arthritis deformans, iritis and iridocyclitis rheumatics, dermatoses.

What is especially valuable about his book for practitioners is that he addresses as well the topic of what conditions do not respond well to bee venom therapy.

Some ethical questions regarding bee sting applications

You have to know that once the bee stings you, she will die within a few hours, as her sting apparatus has been ruptured. This may seem cruel at first glance.

As a beekeeper I am used to the fact – though I'm very careful – that I crush some bees unwittingly when taking out and putting back the frames when handling my hives.

Taking into account that I'm helping my bees when I handle my hives and considering that not the bee but the whole colony is the organism, the unit that has to survive and stay safe, unintentionally crushing some bees is a kind of compromise.

But no compromise should be used as an excuse for exploitation. The bees should be honored and we should be grateful for each gift we receive from them, be it healing or bee products. This attitude could be compared to that of many tribal people. They were hunters but they revered and were grateful to the spirit of the hunted animals. They didn't hunt for profit, but for their everyday survival.

For some it may seem ridiculous, but before applying bee stings I light a wax candle and put the box with bees close to it and I thank the bees for their healing gift.

Success stories with bee venom

Since the days of Dr. Philip Terc and Dr. Bodog F. Beck, lots of cases with positive outcomes have been described.

I will mention here two recently published success stories. The first is that of Ellie Lobel who had already given up her struggle when suddenly an accident happened which changed her life and the course of her illness. The other story of Vanessa Youness shows how structured phyto-apitherapy, lifestyle changes and improved sleep patterns may change the advance of an incurable disease.

Lyme-disease

Maybe the most interesting story is that of Ellie Lobel, whose book *Bee Venom therapy for Lyme-Disease* just has been published.

Ellie was 27 when she got infected with Lyme disease. This condition is caused by a corkscrew-shaped bacteria (Borrelia burgdorfer) which enters the body via tick bites.

She didn't recognize the symptom, the "bull's eye" after being bitten. Ellie thought it was just a strange spider bite. Then flu-like symptoms and horrific pains followed for some months. She wasn't able to get up from her bed.

Physicians she went to gave her different diagnoses: Multiple sclerosis, Fibromyalgia, Rheumatoid arthritis, Lupus.

A proper diagnosis came only a year after she got infected. But it was too late.

The problem with Lyme disease is that Borrelia can persist in the human body. A recent study clearly demonstrates that autopsy tissue sections of the heart, brain, liver and kidney in a Lyme-disease patient treated with antibiotics showed significant pathological changes, including borrelial spirochetal clusters. Moreover the aggregates had alginate, a biofilm marker, on their surfaces, signifying they are true biofilm.[59]

> *The bacteria causing Lyme disease can live in different organs of the body, even in the brain, causing neurological symptoms in the patients.*

That means that although a cure with antibiotics can be applied, the bacteria is capable of hiding in the body's organs. As soon as one stops the antibiotics, the bacteria bounce back.

Ellie just kept doing different treatments but her ailment was continuously worsening. She got stuck in a wheelchair and felt as if she'd lost her short-term memory. She wasn't either able to think clearly. Ellie tried every medicine, antibiotic and treatment available against Lyme-disease.

With some things she would get better for a while, and then she would just relapse right back into her horrible nightmare.

In the following fifteen years she spent all her money and was going broke without experiencing any lasting improvement for her aggravated and torturing disease.

Ellie was prepared and ready to die. She made the decision to move to California and wait for her death there. She knew she would die within the next few months.

Three days after moving something happened that made her think she would die much earlier than expected.

She was attacked by Africanized bees when going out to get some fresh air with her caregiver.

When the bees attacked them, her caregiver ran away but Ellie couldn't even walk. She could more or less hide her eyes and mouth from the stings.

In that moment she was sure she would die because as a small child, at age two, had been stung by a bee and that had nearly killed her. They had to revive her at the hospital with defibrillation. Since then she had avoided bees.

But after a while the swarm flew away leaving her alone.

When the returning caregiver wanted to take her to the hospital, she refused. She saw the attack as "God's way" of putting her out of her misery.

She isolated herself in her room and told her helper to come and collect her body the next day. However, even though she was tormented by awful pains a few hours later, she survived.

These pains weren't a part of a hyper-allergic reaction, as Ellie later realized, but rather a so called Jarisch–Herxheimer response: her body was swamped with toxins from the dead bacteria.

In three days, her pains disappeared and she felt the "brain fog" that was caused by Lyme-disease lift for the first time in years.

Ellie tried to find out what had actually happened to her and why she got better.

But she only found a small study back in 1997 done by researchers from Rocky Mountain Laboratories which described that melittin, the most important compound in bee venom inhibited the growth of the bacteria Borrelia in vitro. Upon closer inspection, the researchers realized that the bacteria were paralyzed and their membranes fell apart as an effect of the melittin.[60]

Though this was scarce information, Ellie was convinced that due to the accident with the Africanized bees she had experienced all this in vivo.

She started to keep bees in her flat and applied bee stings to herself three days a week, 10 stings/session. After three years and many thousands of stings she seemed to be in very good health. Now she has bees on hand for emergency cases, but she doesn't need any stings for her Lyme-disease.

Multiple Sclerosis

In Dr. Stefan Stangaciu's[i] recently published book (not yet available in English)[ii], we find the success story of Vanessa Youness, a patient with multiple sclerosis.

---

i Apitherapist in Europe, author of several books on apitherapy, president of the German Apitherapy Society.

ii Dr. Stefan Stangaciu, Dr. Vanessa Youness, Tratamentul Pas cu Pasul Al Sclerozei Multiplei Prin Apiterapie, Isbn 978-973-0-29255-8, Bucuresti, 2019;

The book provides important information and valuable documentation on phyto- and apitherapy (including bee venom therapy), confirming that this form of treatment, along with lifestyle and dietary changes and improved sleep patterns, are effective against serious diseases.

In Latin, the term **multiple sclerosis** (MS) means many scars (plaques/lesions), which develop on the spinal cord and white matter of the brain during the disease.

MS is the most common immune disorder in which the insulating covers (myelin) of nerve cells in the spinal cord and brain are damaged.

As a result, parts of the nervous system fail to transmit signals. The causes aren't clear yet. They may include genetics, environmental factors being triggered by viral infections etc.

The mechanism is believed to be either destruction by the immune system or failure of the cells producing myelin.

Symptoms can include muscle weakness, trouble with coordination and sensation, double vision, blindness in one eye etc.

Symptoms may occur either in isolated attacks or progressively, building up over time. Symptoms may disappear completely between attacks, but neurological issues persist with the advance of the illness. Worldwide there are about 2.5-3 million people affected by MS.

Vanessa Youness was diagnosed with the disease at the age of 22 after she lost consciousness and collapsed. She was given interferon, a treatment for relapsing multiple sclerosis.

Initially, she didn't accept the diagnosis and visited two other clinics in two different countries (Italy and Britain) to get it confirmed.

Unfortunately, the first diagnosis from her home country, Romania, was corroborated by the next two.

So she had to acknowledge the diagnosis and the fact that she had an incurable disease.

After pondering her options with interferon, she turned to Dr. Stangaciu who was recommended to her by one of her friends.

The phyto-apitherapy the young lady received was a structured one, consisting of mental, emotional, and physical recommendations and cures.

Relaxing mental techniques were (as described in the book):

- Swimming,

- Yoga,

- Tai-Chi,

- Pilates,

- Wim Hof respiration,

- Martial arts,

- Meditation;

For the emotional and spiritual treatment she used:

- infused plants,

- infusion and tincture of leaves and St John's wort which effectively relaxes the nervous system;

- infused root of valerian;

- infused rosemary before bedtime for a calm sleep;

- infused lavender flowers also at bedtime for a calm sleep;

She also had good experiences with:

- tinctures of lavender, arnica and valerian;

- pulverized linden flower and nettle leaves;

- massage oils, sea-buckthorn-, jasmine-, geranium-, ginger- and lemon-balm, sage-oil;

- diffused natural oils in the room (lavender, rose, jasmine, cypress, bergamot and mint) for in the room;

For the physical treatment she took bee products:

- ground bee bread of dog rose;

- ground pollen;

- propolis tincture without alcohol;

- two teaspoons of royal jelly and honey before meals – 3x a day – (a 3 month treatment, followed by a one month break before beginning the treatment again) A bee venom therapy was added to this one.

She also learned the importance of relaxing sleep and lifestyle and dietary changes.

Following the recommendations and the treatment of Dr. Stangaciu, Vanessa Youness got annual MRIs to document how her disease progresses. But the five year analysis confirmed that her MS hadn't advanced. The 4 lesions she was diagnosed with had started to crystallize and didn't cause any further symptoms.

A promising innovation – fighting HIV

Researchers from the Washington University in St. Louis have found that nanoparticles loaded with melittin (the key compound in bee venom) are capable of destroying the human immunodeficiency virus (HIV) while leaving the body's cells unharmed.[61]

Melittin can break through the protective envelope that surrounds viruses like HIV. Besides being able to fight viruses, research has also shown that melittin is an effective tumor-cell killer.

Actually, bee venom or any toxin in it wasn't used to treat chronic diseases in the clinical environment, as it was found that it also harms other human cells.

But nanoparticles do not harm normal cells. And that's a real innovation: the research team engineered protective bumpers to the nanoparticles' surface so that the particles safely bounce off when they come in contact with larger body cells.

Since viruses are much smaller than the nanoparticle they slip between the bumpers, allowing melittin to access the virus.

According to the researchers, this method differs from the way that most anti-HIV drugs work, as they inhibit the virus's ability to reproduce. But this drug does not end the actual infection and there are strains that reproduce anyway.

The melittin loaded on nanoparticles attacks an inherent physical property of the virus and, in theory, there is no way for the virus to adapt to that.

The new nanoparticle delivery mechanism was developed for other purposes and experiments. The nanoparticles were used as an artificial blood product. Though they didn't work well for delivering oxygen, they circulate safely in the body and can serve for the delivery of melittin.

The researchers are hoping that the nanoparticle delivery mechanism can be applied in fighting other viruses as well, as they have the same kind of protective envelope.

Bee venom, propolis, an antibiotic proposed for treatments to fight the coronavirus?

In a Chinese study, 5115 beekeepers were surveyed from February 23 to March 8 (2020), including 723 in Wuhan, the outbreak epicentre of COVID-19. None of these beekeepers developed symptoms associated with the coronavirus, and their health was normal. The researchers also interviewed five apitherapists in Wuhan and followed 121 patients of their apitherapy clinic. These patients had received bee venom therapy in an earlier month, and all the five bee apitherapists use bee venom themselves to treat or prevent certain diseases. Without any protective measures, two of the five apitherapists were exposed to suspected coronavirus cases and others were exposed to confirmed COVID-19 cases, but none of them were infected. None of the 121 patients were infected by the coronavirus, and three of them had close contact with immediate family members who were confirmed SARS-CoV-2 infection cases.[62]

Well, there are open questions regarding these cases and researchers in Germany and other countries also launched their own interviews regarding the beekeepers immunity to the coronavirus.

But another paper (in preprint) written by Dr. Janice Block MD proposes the use of propolis, bee venom and/or azithromycin (a widely used antibiotic) as a preventative measure for individuals at high risk for serious coronavirus infection.[63]

Dr. Janice Block stresses that since both azithromycin and bee-derived products, like propolis, compete against mechanisms by which the virus "opens the door" to the respiratory system, they seem to be excellent choices in the prevention.

Azithromycin is a well-known antibiotic used for the treatment of a number of bacterial infections, including strep throat, middle ear infections, pneumonia, traveler's diarrhea, intestinal infections, etc.

This antibiotic is already in use in the recent pandemic as it protects the epithelial[i] barrier function of the lungs.

Propolis and bee venom could be of potential use as well, both on account of their anti-inflammatory properties and also due to their antimicrobial properties.

There are 3 reasons why azithromicyn, bee-derived products might work well:

1. Azithromycin and bee-derived products appear to be capable of protecting epithelial tight junctions[ii].

---

i Epithelial tissues line the outer surfaces of organs and blood vessels throughout the body, as well as the inner surfaces of cavities in many internal organs. An example is the epidermis, the outermost layer of the skin.

ii Tight junctions seal adjacent epithelial cells in a narrow band just beneath their apical surface. They consist of a network of claudins and other proteins.

2. Reactivation of the coronavirus infection may involve the matrikine[i] PGP[ii] or its derivatives, especially in individuals with chronic lung disease or other risk factors. Azithromycin is promising as a prophylactic agent in post-infection prevention.

3. The most serious cases appear to involve a cytokine[iii] storm, a potentially deadly complication. Azithromycin and bee products modulate this inflammatory response.

Let's see in detail:

Epithelial intercellular tight junctions prevent the invasion of pathogenic bacteria.

Coronaviruses may target epithelial tight junctions, just as other viral pathogens do.

Dr. Janice Block writes, "Though it is not yet known whether the coronavirus participates directly in the degradation of epithelial tight junctions, it's known that it promotes the secretion of cytokines (TNF-alpha and IFN-gamma), that have been associated with increases in barrier dysfunction and mislocalization of tight junction proteins."

In contrast to this, azithromycin displays a sealing effect on respiratory tight junctions. This is independent of its antimicrobial effects.

Brazilian Green Propolis was found to rescue mislocalized proteins (claudin1) in a keratinocyte-derived cell line.[iv] That means compounds of propolis exhibit sealant effects on epithelial tight junctions as well.

Tight junctions perform two vital functions: They limit the passage of molecules and ions through the space between cells.

i Extracellular peptides (matrix-derived) which regulate cell activity.

ii The tripeptide Proline-Glycine-Proline (PGP) is a collagen-derived matrikine.

iii Cytokines are small proteins especially important in the immune system; cytokines modulate the balance between humoral and cell-based immune responses.

iv Single-cell keratinocyte cultures are the most simple in vitro cell culture models available that mimic the epidermal layer of the skin.

When it comes to epithelial tight junctional integrity, young people may have an advantage. They might have more tight junction-sealing proteins (claudins), which might account for their decreased susceptibility to the coronavirus.

An additional concern for older people is that oral pathogens could also lead to a decrease in tight junctional integrity.

Aging leads to hyposalivation in the oral cavity, which affects the composition of oral flora and causes the growth of candida species.

By interfering with the epithelial barrier of the oropharynx, *Candida albicans* might facilitate the penetration of coronaviruses from the upper respiratory tract.

Another potential challenge to tight junctional integrity of the upper airway is *Porphyromonas gingivalis*, an oral pathogen related to periodontitis.[i]

Gum disease caused by *P. gingivalis* has been shown to respond to treatment by both bee venom and azithromycin.

Azithromycin kills *P. gingivalis*; and it has been shown to reduce pro-inflammatory cytokines induced by *P. gingivalis* LPS

Bee venom has also been found to inhibit pro-inflammatory cytokines induced by P. gingivalis.

Reactivation of coronavirus infection may involve the matrikine PGP or its derivatives. PGP, a pro-inflammatory compound that can worsen risk in individuals with COPD[ii] or respiratory-associated sepsis, has been shown to be modulated by azithromycin in individuals with COPD.

Thus, azithromycin is promising as a prophylactic agent in post-infection prevention, particularly in the context of COPD or other chronic lung disease.

---

i Also called gum disease.

ii Chronic Obstructive Pulmonary Disease (COPD) The main symptoms: shortness of breath and cough with sputum production. It is a progressive disease and it typically worsens over time.

It is believed that the greatest danger with the coronavirus is in part due to the cytokine storm, an exaggerated release of inflammatory cytokines, which leads to respiratory system failure.

In addition to azithromycin, melittin, an anti-inflammatory compound derived from bee venom, reduces the formation of such cytokines.

The anti-inflammatory cytokine IL10 downregulates inflammatory cytokines such as IL1 and TNF alpha. IL10 has been associated with improved outcomes, both in animal models of LPS associated sepsis and also in coronavirus infections.

Increases in IL10 are expected to play a protective role both by attenuating cytokine storm, and also by strengthening epithelial barrier function. By reducing TNF alpha, IL10 likely exerts an (indirect) protective effect on TER and on respiratory epithelial tight junctions, thus preventing further invasion by viral particles.

Interestingly, beekeepers have increased IL10 compared to the general population. Presumably this increase relates to exposure to bee venom. Beekeepers are probably protected to some significant degree against the worst of the pandemic. Obviously it does not mean that they do not need social distancing or other protective measures.

This observation suggests that, in individuals at high risk, prophylaxis with bee venom or with active ingredients contained in bee venom might be able to prevent or attenuate cytokine storm in the context of the recent pandemic.

However while further research is needed to isolate effective active ingredients from these bee products to limit potential complications, bee-derived products have the great advantage of not carrying the risk of increased antibiotic resistance.

Considering all the reasons above, Dr. Janice Block proposes azithromycin , bee venom and propolis as preventative measures for individuals at high risk for serious coronavirus infection.

You can read the original paper by Dr. Janice Block here: https://www.researchgate.net/publication/340398571

Summary

- Adrenal glands stimulated by the bee venom release cortisol.

- Melittin in bee venom has an anti-inflammatory activity and it can break through the protective envelope that surrounds viruses.

- No alcohol or antihistamines should be used during bee venom therapy.

- One of the goals of bee venom therapy is to stimulate the immune system.

- A kit containing epinephrine is a must!

- No effects of bee venom: a sign that it will work.

- About one to two percent of the population is hyper-allergic to bee venom.

- It's important to realize the difference between the normal effects and hyper-allergy.

- Bee Venom Immunotherapy is advised for hyper-allergic persons.

- Bee venom can be also administered by injection or as a cream. A meridian massage with a cream containing bee venom can be very effective.

- A successful therapy for chronic diseases, should consist of mental, emotional, and physical recommendations and cures.

- Researchers found that nanoparticles loaded with melittin are capable of destroying the human immunodeficiency virus (HIV) while leaving the body's cells unharmed.

- A physician proposes azithromycin, bee venom and propolis as preventative measures for individuals at high risk of serious coronavirus infection.

What about other bee products?

Although you can read about the use of pollen and royal jelly in the interview with Dr. Stangaciu in this book, you may also ask why I don't write about these bee products in more detail.

First, though I have some experience with them, I do not have as much as with honey, propolis or bee venom.

On the other hand, some of the other bee products e.g. royal jelly, can't be kept easily in a home pharmacy: it must be fresh or kept in the fridge to experience its benefits.

> *Then, in my opinion, it isn't ethical to take some bee products from the bees – bee bread, for instance, serves as the basic nutrient- (proteins, minerals etc.) rich food for the bees.*

You may say that honey also serves as a basic food for the bees and you take it. While this is true, I take about one third or maximum half of it, if my bees collect it in abundance.

Plus, honey is not actually the basic food for the bees. Rather, it's a source of carbohydrates they use for heating and energy supply. As I don't feed sugar syrup to my bees, before each honey extraction in the summer, I assess how much honey should be left for them to survive the winter if no more nectar could be collected before winter.

Royal jelly

As a beekeeper, I eat this regularly in spring, when there are some queen cells in my hives and I do some swarm control or handle my hives. But I don't harvest royal jelly systematically and I don't keep it in my home pharmacy as its harvesting requires special procedures and tools and it should be kept in the fridge.

Royal jelly is actually the enzyme secreted from the glands in the heads of the bees. The worker bees feed royal jelly to the queen larvae.

It is actually the queen-maker as its composition determines which bee larvae will develop into a queen. The jelly the bees feed to the drones or worker bees is a bit different.

Royal jelly has a sour taste and usually 3x1-2 grams is advised to be consumed by patients. When I overeat it when handling my hives, it causes some belly pain and diarrhea.

It's believed that it has an immunostimulating effect and a lot of other benefits: antiaging, fertility boosting, reducing menopause syndromes, lowering blood pressure, regulating blood sugar, supporting brain functions, increasing tear secretion etc.

As its use may have adverse effects (vomiting, diarrhea, wheezing, nausea etc.), and it may also interact with some drugs, such as blood pressure drugs, it is best to contact a specialist who will integrate it into your apitherapy.

Pollen and bee bread

Pollen is the protein and other nutrient source for the bees. Honey bees collect it from spring to fall and store it as bee bread. Pollen is taken by beekeepers with different types of pollen collectors when the bees bring it to their hives.

Pollen is believed to be a good food supplement, as it contains nutrients, vitamins, amino acids, lipids and over 250 active substances.

It is important to know that pollen can't be digested by the bees or humans in raw form as its outer layer consists of a highly decay-resistant chemical called sporopollenin. Grinding it is not easy either, as it requires a very special grinder. That's why the bees mix the pollen with honey and some lactobacteria to ferment it.

In my opinion, the collection of pollen can be ethical only if the beekeeper takes care not to take large amounts of pollen from the bees, I'd say a maximum of 15%.

Lacking the protein and different nutrients from the bee bread can result in high susceptibility to diseases in bees.

Trying to use pollen (be it in shakes or coffee) caused diarrhea and bloating for me. That's why I avoid it. A good apitherapist could help with these issues and control the correct intake or integrate its use into apitherapy sessions.

On the other hand, bee bread (the fermented pollen) can be easily digested and it seems to be a great pre- and probiotic (containing lactobacteria). I sometimes eat a bit of it when handling my hives. Or when a colony doesn't survive the winter and there is some bee bread left. I take out the combs containing it and pull out the small pieces of bee bread from the cells with a pin. You can imagine that this is a very time consuming harvest. But, all in all, I think it's not ethical to take bee bread from the honey bees.

A kind of bee bread can be made by the beekeeper, too, by mixing pollen and honey and letting this mixture "ripen".

Hive air

Recently, some beekeepers have offered hive air in bee houses where you can relax and enjoy the benefits of the volatile compounds of propolis, wax, honey, bees, and pollen. Hive air is relaxing and it can be helpful for different lung diseases. It is absolutely contraindicated with allergies to pollen or bee venom.

However, I inhale some hive air from the small observation hive I use for educational purposes I just have designed a small mobile bee house where my wife and I will be able to sleep as well. I'm building it right now and I'm looking forward to using it in the very near future.

Prof. Dr. Eberhart Bengsche from the Max Planck Institute in Munich, lists the following conditions that can be helped with hive air:

Bronchitis

Asthma

Allergy

Pseudocrope (false diphtheria)

COPD (chronic obstructive pulmonary inflammation, susceptibility to infection, chronic inflammation that leads to the development of tumors.

Immune system weakening

Chronic headaches, migraine

Depression.

Summary

- The worker bees feed royal jelly to the queen larvae.

- It's believed that it has an immunostimulating effect and a lot of other benefits: antiaging, fertility boosting, reducing menopause syndromes, lowering blood pressure, regulating blood sugar, supporting brain functions, increasing tear secretion.

- Pollen is the protein source for the bees.

- Pollen is a good food supplement, as it contains nutrients, vitamins, amino acids, lipids and over 250 active substances.

- Honey is a source of carbohydrates they use for heating and energy supply.

- A kind of bee bread can be made by the beekeeper, too, by mixing pollen and honey and letting this mixture "ripen".

- Hive air is relaxing and it can be helpful for different lung diseases.

11. KEEPING BEES IN AN OBSERVATION HIVE

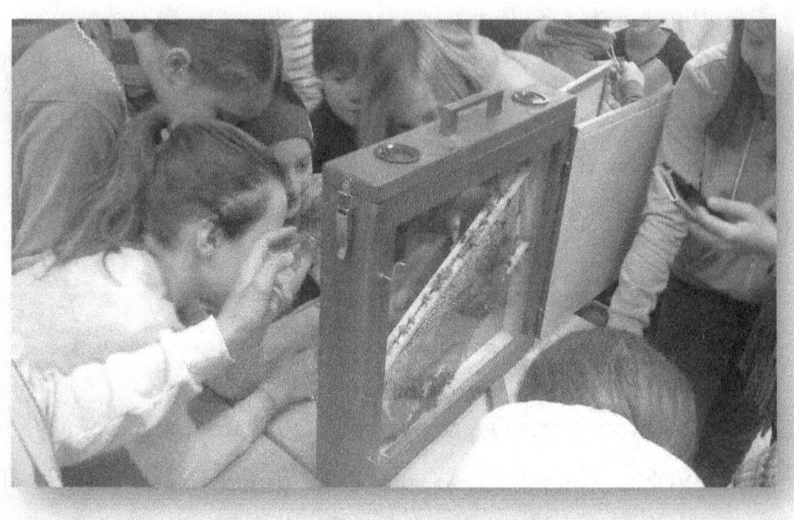

In this section you'll learn:

- How to keep bees in an observation hive;

- The parameters of a small hive;

- About an app and a card game, if you wish to know more about bees;

Bees in the observational hive

As a teacher, I use a small hive in the classroom when teaching about bees to let my pupils watch the bees, queen, larvae, eggs, honey, pollen, and different phenomena, like dancing or clustering of the bees to build the wax comb etc.

This small hive has the capacity of one frame and can be home to 2-3000 bees, a queen and 50-100 drones. Its two walls are made of hardened glass. As the bees don't like being exposed to light this small hive can be darkened or shadowed on the sides by two wooden boards on hinges. Kids love watching bees, just as I do.

Most of the time I keep this observation hive in my office, near my desk. Not only is watching the bees an uplifting experience for me, but so is smelling them. The small hive has two holes on the top, closed by plastic mesh, where I can feed them, if necessary. And through these holes I can smell the fragrance of the honey and pollen.

The fragrance changes from one day to another depending on the nectar varietal the bees have just collected. It's always a surprise to smell what the fragrance will be. Sometimes it fills the whole room, when the bees ventilate hard to dry the nectar and turn it into honey.

When the weather is nice and I don't need the observation hive for the classroom, I take it outside and let the bees fly out. If they are confined for several days I check their food stock in the comb and if necessary I feed them with some honey or sugar syrup.

If there is no water in the area I give them some water through the plastic mesh.

This small hive is useful when it comes to applying bee stings as well, just as you have seen in the story about curing my aggravated flu with bee stings.

I only keep a frame of bees in the observational hive for 2-3 weeks, then I put it back into the colony I've initially taken them from and, if needed for educational purposes or therapy, I take out another frame full of bees.

I do this because a small unit of bees – which is the small colony in the observational hive- does not feel very comfortable being separated from its original home: It can become more susceptible to pests and its capacity for organizing itself is also reduced.

The observation hive should:

> - be portable;
>
> - be stable when put down on a table or the ground;
>
> - be made of hardened glass on both sides for security reasons;
>
> - be easily disassembled with a power screwdriver for proper cleaning; (when cleaning it, take care handling the glass as it can cut you or get broken;)
>
> - have holes closed with plastic or wire mesh on the top so that you can feed the bees easily.

You can get bees on frames from beekeepers or order bee packages. I think it is best to contact a local beekeeper.

Responsibility and precautions

Keeping bees involves responsibility for the bees, yourself, your family and other people living with you or for your neighbors. I do not encourage anyone to keep bees in an observational hive without beekeeping knowledge or experience. I only describe how I keep them in the observational hive in my office, in addition to my apiary.

Precautions I take:

> I handle the hive and the bees very carefully;
>
> I don't leave kids alone when watching the bees in the observational hive in the classroom;
>
> I make sure to place the hive where no one can drop it or kick it by accident.
>
> Epinephrine injection and alcohol is available when applying bee stings.

Taking care of the bees in the observational hive:

I take the small hive outside and let the bees fly out from time to time (at least twice a week) as they need to clear their digestive system and collect nectar and pollen. I make sure they aren't disturbing my neighbors. When clearing their digestive systems, they may make the clothes on the line messy!

Before returning the observation hive to the room, I wait until all the bees are back in the hive. Once they have discovered nectar or pollen in the area, they can work until dusk;

If their food stock is low, I feed them with honey or sugar syrup. If the bees won't be returned to their original colony later they can be fed with honey, but beekeepers don't usually feed honey to bees as this can support the spread of foulbrood spores, a dangerous pest of the bee brood; Sugar syrup can be easily made by mixing a 1:1 ratio of sugar and lukewarm water;

I dissemble the observational hive (without bees!) and clean it at least twice a year;

When keeping bees in the observational hive over the winter I take care that they are kept at 5 to 7 °C in a cellar or cool pantry with a large enough honey supply in the combs. And when the weather makes it possible in the spring, I let them fly out;

When taking the observational hive outside in the early spring, I make sure not to leave it there overnight as the temperature may go down. The bees may use up all of their honey stock in the small colony and "freeze" by morning.

If this happens and I find the bees motionless in the small hive the next morning, I take out the frame and sprinkle the bees with diluted honey or sugar syrup. They may come to life even if they looked dead before. Precaution is needed when taking out and replacing the frame.

Lessons about bees

It all began with a question from my son when I was showing him around in a hive and we tried to find the queen.

He asked, "Isn't there any bee game through which we could play and learn about bees?"

Later, I was looking for such games and I didn't find any. My son said bee cards or an app would be a great way to teach him about bees.

After some brainstorming, we decided to create a bee version of the classic deck of cards.

We started to take pictures in our apiary and to design the cards. Through our common project we learned about patience and perseverance, trial and error. The wonderful thing is, we actually turned his idea into a unique product that works! And we've also completed beeQuiz, an educational application.

Then a few years ago I decided to offer lessons about bees in schools. I've built up a complex curriculum to introduce bees to children. And it turned out that kids are truly amazed by the wonderful lives of bees. We learn about them through real time observation, art, and lots of games. While having fun we incidentally learn that nature and our environment is worthy of our respect! And we use Bee Cards and the beeQuiz app as well. They are actually the most successful elements of my bee lessons.

If you'd like to know more about honey bees I recommend the Bee Cards and the beeQuiz app. We are working on the international English versions of the app and the card game and we hope they will be soon available internationally. You can visit the site www.healer-bees.com to find information about the project.

Summary

- An observational hive is useful for educational goals and when it comes to applying bee stings.

- Keeping bees involves responsibility for the bees, yourself, your family and your neighbors.

- Take it outside whenever it's possible and let the bees fly out.
- Check their food stock in the comb and if necessary feed them with some honey or sugar syrup.

- Before returning the observation hive to the room, wait until all the bees are back in the hive.

- Dissemble the observational hive (without bees!) and clean it at least twice a year;

- When keeping bees in the observational hive over the winter take care that they are kept at 5° to 7°C (41° to 44°F)in a cellar or cool pantry with a large enough honey supply in the combs.

- When taking the observational hive outside in the early spring, make sure not to leave it there overnight as the temperature may go down.

- Precaution is needed when taking out and replacing the frame.

- Bee Cards and beeQuiz – useful tools to learn about bees.

12. MAKING LIFESTYLE CHANGES

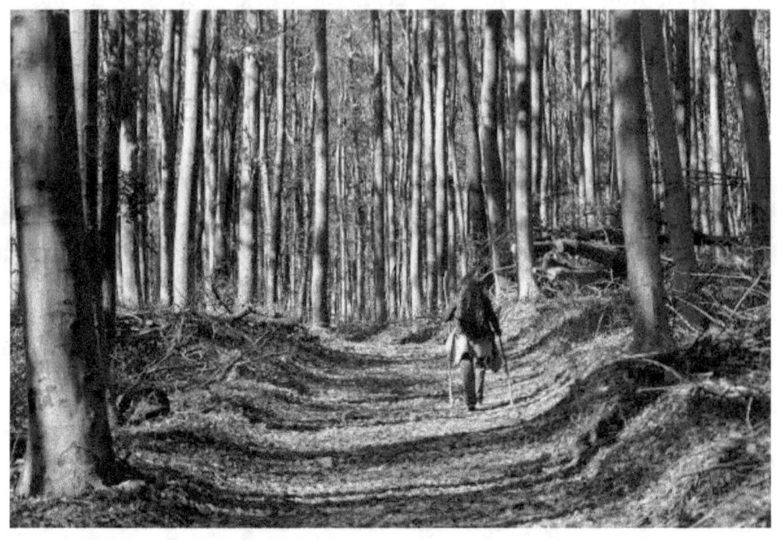

In this section you'll learn:

- How to make lifestyle changes by knowing yourself;

- About testing and keeping what is good for you;

- A retrospective analysis;

Why are lifestyle choices so difficult to make?

It would be so nice to reduce sugary food or quit nicotine, alcohol, too much caffeine etc., to move regularly or to do exercise, so that we can prevent or get rid of all health issues.

But lifestyle choices are difficult to make. We can make New Year's resolutions or we can decide to change some of our bad habits.

Usually these decisions don't happen at a deeper level, so we only follow them for a while, but not long-term.

One of the reasons may be that some unconscious impulses drive us, be it some forgotten childhood events – they don't necessarily need to be traumatizing ones- be it of other origins.

But, of course, there are many methods to bring more light to our unconsciousness: different psychological systems: family systems, transactional analyses etc.)

I think our common sense can also help. Simply by looking for the reasons and asking questions when something, for instance a health issue, comes up, can bring some light into this area. (See *How to find out the causes of our disorders, page 36*)

The other reason why New Year's resolutions don't work is that avoiding a bad habit or food is not enough, we have to do something instead, otherwise the space left behind can make us feel bad and we'll fill the space again with the same habit or food.

But with both of the above issues – unconscious impulses, the void after dropping a bad habit- understanding of the following can help.

Know yourself

I hope you'll find the following thoughts useful when making your own lifestyle choices and changes. So, I invite you to think about them and "hold on to what is good" for you.

We're told several times each day on ad boards, radio, tv, social media etc., that we are individuals and we are unique. We tend to believe this without thinking about it too much.

But the media message isn't meant to have you think about your uniqueness either, its only goal is to flatter you and to draw your attention to a stylish product they want you to buy.

Ironically, the fact is that you really are unique.

> *One of the main and interesting tasks is to "know yourself", even if this constant process never ends.*

As I am talking in this book about health issues, let me explain from this point of view.

You may have tried many lifestyle choices, such as vegetarianism, veganism, gluten-free, low-carb, keto or paleo diet, different sports, exercises, methods etc.

The experience may be that any lifestyle change will work and get good results for a while. It may even work for a longer period, like a decade, but then you may have the experience that something went wrong and you don't feel comfortable you have to give up some habits and engage new ones.

Why is this? Well, actually it is because you are an individual and you are unique, as are the situations you are involved in.

A lifestyle (veganism, paleo diet etc.) may work for 80-90% of people very well, even for you. But what if you are in the 10-20%?

Besides the task of "know yourself", the other task is "Test them all and hold on to what is good".

"Test them all and hold on to what is good"

My grandfather, to whom I dedicated this book, once told me in my adolescence, when I was making fun of the town's idiot, that I should listen to this strange guy respectfully, because one never knows where important life messages come from. "Then using your common sense, you can make your choice."

It was yet another great lesson from my grandfather that I am thankful for.

This applies to lifestyle changes, practices and methods as well.

I'm grateful to fate that I have had the chance to try many lifestyle choices, diets, sports, arts, jobs etc. I know each has enriched or can enrich my life in one way or another, and I know everything I was enthusiastic about and I tried or practiced for shorter or longer times has brought important things into my life.

But learning for life sometimes involves giving up things as well: particularly when we realize they don't work anymore. I don't want to say that we should give things up as soon as we feel uncomfortable with them. Perseverance is important. But when we realize that they are damaging or endangering our lives, we should skip them or rethink what we can retain from them. I'm sure it wasn't an accident they came our way.

In many cases, our enthusiasm or established habits make us blind to the damage some lifestyle choices can cause.

Again, I don't want to tell you what is a good health or lifestyle habit for you, because what is good for me may harm you and everything you get engaged in and practice will bring some good to you!

You have to be ready to act and make your own choices to give up things but retain what is good for you.

As life itself is a constant flow, health doesn't seem to be stagnant either. That's another reason that a single lifestyle choice won't guarantee wellbeing and health for your entire life.

An "out-of-the-box" practice to test: the Wim Hof method

Sometimes things cross your path that are worth trying out, and if they work well then you keep them for your own needs. Since I published the first edition of this book, The Wim Hof Method crossed my path.

The method was also used by Vanessa Younnes in her protocol to cure Multiple sclerosis, as mentioned earlier in this book.

Wim Hof developed his method after a family drama and broke many records of cold exposure, including climbing Mount Everest only in shorts and boots or running a half marathon barefoot on snow and ice, swimming under the ice etc.

The Wim Hof Method consists of respiratory exercises, exposure to cold and meditation.

While being investigated scientifically, it turned out that through his self-developed method he was able to reduce inflammation when administered an endotoxin (*Escherichia coli*) in his blood.

The scientists wanted to know whether this was only a special ability of Wim Hof or if the observation could be repeated with other individuals trained in the method.

Wim Hof trained a group for 10 days and the experiment was repeated with those people, too.[64]

The experiment showed that the trained people who were practicing the method and were administered the endotoxin had elevated levels of epinephrine and cytokine Il-10. IL 10 downregulates proinflammatory cytokines, as you may remember from an earlier chapter in this book, "Bee venom, propolis and antibiotics proposed for treatments to fight the coronavirus". Beekeepers exposed to bee-stings regularly have elevated levels of IL-10.

This information and common feature with bee sting therapy convinced me to try the method.

> *After doing 3-4 rounds of Wim Hof respiratory exercises[i], the blood becomes more alkaline, from pH 7.4 to 7.75, but then returns in the post exercise period.*

---

[i] One round consists of 30 breathes, inhaling fully, then letting the air out (not pressing it fully out, just as the lungs would do it). At the last exhalation the breath should be retained for as long as one can (1-3 or more minutes). When now one feels the need to inhale, he or she inhales fully and retains the breath for 15 seconds. Then the next round follows.

A very interesting and, somewhat alarming result, was that in the experiment, after the rounds, oxygen saturation went down significantly when the subjects held their breath. After the third breathing round it may drop to about 50 %, but it goes back right after the normalization of breathing.

The method undoubtedly has its physical benefits. But those tuned for spiritual experiences will learn a lot about themselves, their willpower, motivation or some of their hidden psychological aspects.

In the retention phase of Wim Hof breathing, especially after 3-4 rounds, one may experience stroboscopic images or sensations. I reckon this happens because as the oxygen level goes down for a short time endocannabinoids are released in the brain.

If you are a chronic disease-free person, you may try the method.

However, it is to be mentioned that being aware of our body's signs is very important when practicing the WHM and that overdoing exposure to cold or the respiratory exercises may also be harmful. Therefore, besides mastering our willpower – without that resisting a cold shower isn't possible – is necessary to listen to our body's signs and, if needed, to stop practicing cold exposure until we are fit again.

Some people practicing the method for longer claim that they developed a kind of addiction to it. I know some others who did sports intensively and in parallel to that also took cold showers twice a day claim that they developed joint pains. Again: overdoing it for any reason, whether it be for raising performance or because you've experienced the benefits of it isn't good!

After 4 months of daily practice, now I do it twice or three times a week which is comfortable and fits into my schedule and with my health condition.

I mention the Wim Hof Method as it has some impact on our bodies that share remarkable common features with some apitherapeutic procedures and it is possible to combine them.

The Wim Hof breath can be practiced when inhaling hive air and I assure you it is an extraordinary experience. I have tried it a few times with my observational hive.

At the moment I'm working on my bee mobile house in which we'll be able to directly inhale the air from whole bee colonies. I will report on it in a future article and I'll add it to the next edition of this book, too.

What have you tested and held on to, or what will you?

Lifestyle choices, trends may come and go, but some practices, attitudes and simple insights we have found to be "good" may stay with us. They can be the tools we work with when facing constant changes and building and rebuilding our health.

> *It's worthwhile to think on what are or which ones could be your "tested good practices".*

Yours may differ from mine. If you make a list of lifestyle choices you have made up until now or which you are practicing right now, you may gain an overview of which practices, insights, attitudes are worth keeping and which you don't need any more.

Make a list for yourself; looking at such a "biography" can lead to useful insights. I can only show you a list of what I've taken from the lifestyle choices, diets, sports, and trends that I've tried. In my adolescence I practiced Shotokan exercises, but I didn't carry that into my adult life. Then, two years ago, when I was thinking about viable short exercises to refresh myself during my office work and sooth my back pain while handling my hives, I remembered them. Because I had once loved these exercises, I could integrate them into my life, in contrast to some expert-recommended exercises that I had also tried. These Shotokan exercises weren't something someone had told me to do, they were once already mine.

I just want to stress that nothing comes into our life accidentally. I believe that all things will teach us something. We may integrate them into our life later. But such retrospective surveys can help us to eventually recognize their potential.

All the statements and experiences in the following retrospective list are mine, they are my conclusions, I'm also open to change them when my common sense suggests I should, or when I have a different experience. They may not apply to you. You may find that vegetarianism works very well for you, though unfortunately I had to give it up. It is important to make your own list and search for the solutions to your situation.

Check the sports, diets, lifestyle choices, jobs, beliefs, marriages, partnerships, diseases etc. you have had. Jot down the first 5 that occur to you. Then for each, ask yourself the following questions:

What insights have I gained from it?
What were the advantages of doing/having it?
What practices did I do?
What kept me from it or what is worth retaining from it?
Were there any drawbacks?

My retrospective "lifestyle list" – insights, practices, drawbacks (if there are any);

What I've kept and what I've retained:

From oriental martial sports in my adolescence: I do the basic exercises from Shotokan when working long hours at my desk and I need some refreshing movements; I've also kept the insight from Judo, that everything has an impulse and when "fighting" or even writing, no counterattack or push is needed, just let the oncoming impulses work for me, it is a kind of "go with the flow";

From growing up in a multicultural environment: learning other languages is important and it can be accomplished best and most effectively rereading my favorite books in the foreign language. I learn without using a dictionary and I talk to people even if I'm not fluent in that language. In this way I've learnt several languages.

From a decade of vegetarianism, I kept the oriental spices and recipes I've learnt. The beneficial effects of legumes and fruits.

The importance of fasting in a smart way. But I've also learnt that fasting and vegetarianism can cause insomnia and gallbladder stones for me. (Note: this may differ for other individuals and at different ages!)

From the gluten and milk free diet: I've kept the insight that it can reduce inflammation in the body in an enormous way and when feeling bad because of some infections I stick to this diet for weeks or months.

From paleo diet: though I was a vegetarian for animal friendly reasons I had to accept the fact that eating eggs, meat and fat (not a lot!) is important for my constitution, even though I fought against this insight for some time. The painful experience of gallbladder stones taught me that. the stones went dormant after a few months I changed my diet from vegetarian to paleo. I also hope, that they'll disappear without an operation;

From low carb diet: During "infectious" times I keep away from starchy food to let my self-healing power work at its best; I remove all soft drinks from my diet, even pressed juices, I enjoy eating fruits in their whole form.

From yoga and meditation which I did for some years: I have kept certain assanas (e.g. the Cobra) which also helps me to prevent or sooth my back pain when handling my hives; the insight that slowing down and looking inside can bring peace into agitated moments; the insight that overdoing meditation can distract from everyday life.

From a honey cure for giving up sweets and treating insomnia caused probably by metabolic stress: that honey is a powerful remedy and digesting it is different from "normal" carbohydrates and sugars due to its enzymes, antioxidants, simple sugars, oligosaccharides etc. I retained the habit of a tablespoon of honey at bedtime and one in the morning – when I feel the appetite for it- mostly at 10 a.m.

Well the list may be continued as, especially nowadays, one can try so many things and trends.

Make your own list to confirm your decisions or help you give up habits that aren't good for you anymore.

Summary

- Lifestyle choices are difficult to make. There are many methods to bring more light to our unconsciousness.

- Common sense can also help. Whenever you feel ill look for the reasons and ask the right questions.

- Even if you don't discover the exact cause of a certain pain, nausea etc. this method will make you more conscious of your daily routines.

- Know yourself!

- "Test them all and hold on to what is good"

- Lifestyle choices, trends may come and go, but some practices, attitudes and simple insights you have found to work may stay with you.

Epilogue

When I started to write this book about two years ago I had two health issues that I mentioned at the beginning of this book: backache and periodontitis.

When handling my hives, my backache was very annoying, as it forced me to quit beekeeping for a short time, just as my formal and prompt hypersensitivity to bee venom had done.

By asking the right questions and the retrospective "method" described earlier, I determined the correct exercises to avoid backache. The solution was very simple. I have to do some pushups (25-30 ones) and the cobra asana when handling my hives – all were once part of my life. I would say my backache seems to be completely resolved now.

I've not yet cured my periodontitis, but I have reconsidered and started a treatment with chestnut honey and propolis (washing my gums with them during the day, in the evening I use Paradontax), and bee stings on the right acupuncture points. I'm also regularly consulting a dental surgeon who helped me with this issue by doing periodontal therapy and who is regularly cleaning my dental tartar and plaque.

If you are reading this epilogue it means you've read through this book, for which I'm really grateful!

I hope you have enjoyed *Bees Help Fight Viruses*. If you did, I'd be very grateful if you could write a review. I'd love to hear what you think.

I wish, with all my heart that this book has provided new information, advice and attitudes that you'll take from it and maintain along on your way.

Recommended books:

Bodog F. Beck, (Reprint 1997). The Bible of Bee Venom Therapy;

N. Yoirish, (1977) Curative Properties of Honey and Bee Venom – University Press of the Pacific;

Bogdanov, Stefan. (2016). Honey in Medicine. (available in pdf: https://www.researchgate.net/);

Ron Fessenden, MD. The New Honey Revolution- Kindle E-Book;

Ellie Lobel, (2020). Bee Venom Therapy for Lyme Disease;

Dr. Stefan Stangaciu, Claudette Raynal-Cartabas (2016). En bonne santé avec les abeilles (soon available in English, too);

Lady Cerelli, (2016). Apitherapy - From a Beekeeper's Perspective;

MEDICAL INFORMATION DISCLAIMER

1.   Credit
1.1   This Medical Information Disclaimer was created using a template from SEQ Legal (https://seqlegal.com).
2.   No advice
2.1   This book contains general medical information.
2.2   The medical information is not advice and should not be treated as such.
3.   No warranties
3.1   The medical information in this book is provided without any representations or warranties, express or implied.
3.2   Without limiting the scope of Section 3.1, we do not warrant or represent that the medical information in this book:
(a)   will be constantly available, or available at all; or
(b)   is true, accurate, complete, current or non-misleading.
4.   Medical assistance

4.1   You must not rely on the information in this book as an alternative to medical advice from your doctor or other professional healthcare provider.

4.2   If you have any specific questions about any medical matter, you should consult your doctor or other professional healthcare provider.

4.3   If you think you may be suffering from any medical condition, you should seek immediate medical attention.

4.4   You should never delay seeking medical advice, disregard medical advice or discontinue medical treatment because of information in this book.

5.   Interactive features

5.1   This book includes interactive features that allow users to communicate with the author.

5.2   You acknowledge that, because of the limited nature of communication through the book's interactive features, any assistance you may receive using any such features is likely to be incomplete and may even be misleading.

5.3   Any assistance you may receive using any interactive features does not constitute specific advice and accordingly should not be relied upon without further independent confirmation.

6.   Limits upon exclusions of liability

6.1   Nothing in this disclaimer will:

(a)   limit or exclude any liability for death or personal injury resulting from negligence;

(b)   limit or exclude any liability for fraud or fraudulent misrepresentation;

(c)   limit any liabilities in any way that is not permitted under applicable law; or

(d)   exclude any liabilities that may not be excluded under applicable law.

INDEX

NOTES

PREVENTION

[1] Madas, B.G., Füri, P., Farkas, Á. *et al.* Deposition distribution of the new coronavirus (SARS-CoV-2) in the human airways upon exposure to cough-generated droplets and aerosol particles. *Sci Rep*10, 22430 (2020). https://doi.org/10.1038/s41598-020-79985-6

[2] Baohong Wang, Mingfei Yao, Longxian Lv, Zongxin Ling, Lanjuan Li, The Human Microbiota In Health And Disease, Engineering, Volume 3, Issue 1, 2017, Pages 71-82, ISSN 2095-8099, Https://Doi.Org/10.1016/J.ENG.2017.01.008.

[3] Woolhouse M, Scott F, Hudson Z, Howey R, Chase-Topping M. Human viruses: discovery and emergence. Philos Trans R Soc Lond B Biol Sci. 2012;367(1604):2864–71. doi:10.1098/rstb.2011.0354

[4] Lane JM (2006). "Mass Vaccination And Surveillance/Containment In The Eradication Of Smallpox". Current Topics In Microbiology And Immunology. 304: 17–29. Doi:10.1007/3-540-36583-4_2. ISBN 978-3-540-29382-8. PMC 7120753. PMID 16989262.

[5] Mata, Élida Cleyse Gomes da, Mourão, Caroline Barbosa Farias, Rangel, Marisa, & Schwartz, Elisabeth Ferroni. (2017). Antiviral activity of animal venom peptides and related compounds. Journal of Venomous Animals and Toxins including Tropical Diseases, 23, 3. Epub February 20, 2017.https://dx.doi.org/10.1186/s40409-016-0089-0

6 Meiler F, Zumkehr J, Klinkenberg S, Rucker's B, Akdis CA, Akdis M. In vivo switch to IL10 secreting T regulatory cells in high dose allergen exposure. J Exp Med. 2008, 205: 2887-2898. doi: 10.1084/jet.20080193

[7] Yadav BS, Sharma A, Yadav RB. Studies on effect of multiple heating/cooling cycles on the resistant starch formation in cereals, legumes and tubers. Int J Food Sci Nutr. 2009;60 Suppl 4:258-72. doi: 10.1080/09637480902970975. PMID: 19562607.

[8] Heather F. Smith, William Parker, Sanet H. Kotzé, Michel Laurin. Morphological evolution of the mammalian cecum and cecal appendix. *Comptes Rendus Palevol*, 2017; 16 (1): 39 DOI: 10.1016/j.crpv.2016.06.001

[9] Zhu Y, Yan Y, Gius DR, Vassilopoulos A. Metabolic regulation of Sirtuins upon fasting and the implication for cancer. Curr Opin Oncol. 2013 Nov;25(6):630-6. doi: 10.1097/01.cco.0000432527.49984.a3. PMID: 24048020; PMCID: PMC5525320.

[10] Published in Australasian Beekeeper (2020 issues 11,12) and Hungarian Beekeeping Magazine: Méhészet 2020 issues, 11,12), witten by Mihaly Hevesi

[11] Al-Waili NS.. Natural Honey Lowers Plasma Glucose, C-Reactive Protein, Homocysteine, And Blood Lipids In Healthy, Diabetic, And Hyperlipidemic Subjects: Comparison With Dextrose And Sucrose. J Med Food. 2004 Spring;7(1):100-7

[12] Manning T.S., Gibson G.R. Microbial-Gut Interactions In Health And Disease: Prebiotics. Best Pract. Res. Clin. Gastroenterol. 2004;18:287–298. Doi: 10.1016/J.Bpg.2003.10.008

[13] Kajiwara S., Gandhi H., Ustunol Z. Effect Of Honey On The Growth Of And Acid Production By Human Intestinal Bifidobacterium Spp.: An In Vitro Comparison With Commercial Oligosaccharides And Inulin. J. Food Prot. 2002;65:214–218.

[14] Gibson G.R., Probert H.M., Loo J.V., Rastall R.A., Roberfroid M.B. Dietary Modulation Of The Human Colonic Microbiota: Updating The Concept Of Prebiotics. Nutr. Res. Rev. 2004;17:259–275. Doi: 10.1079/NRR200479

HONEY

[15] Steinberg, D; Kaine, G; Gedalia, I (1996) Antibacterial Effect Of Propolis And Honey On Oral Bacteria. American Journal Of Dentistry 9 (6): 236-239

[16] Ramli NZ, Chin KY, Zarkasi KA, Ahmad F. A Review on the Protective Effects of Honey against Metabolic Syndrome. Nutrients. 2018 Aug 2;10(8):1009. doi: 10.3390/nu10081009. PMID: 30072671; PMCID: PMC6115915.

[17] Larsson SC, Bergkvist L, Wolk A, Consumption Of Sugar And Sugar-Sweetened Foods And The Risk Of Pancreatic Cancer In A Prospective Study. Am J Clin Nutr. 2006 Nov;84(5):1171-6

[18] Fung TT, Malik V, Rexrode KM, Manson JE, Willett WC, Hu FB., Sweetened Beverage Consumption And Risk Of Coronary Heart Disease In Women. Am J Clin Nutr. 2009 Apr;89(4):1037-42. Doi: 10.3945/Ajcn.2008.27140. Epub 2009 Feb 11.

[19] Jenkins, FJ; Wolever, TM; Taylor, RH; Barker, H; Fielden, H; Baldwin, JM; Bowling, AC; Newman, HC; Jenkins, AL; Goff, DF (1981). "Glycemic Index Of Foods: A Physiological Basis For Carbohydrate Exchange". Am J Clin Nutr. 34 (3): 362–6. Doi:10.1093/Ajcn/34.3.362. PMID 6259925.

[20] Deibert P, König D, Kloock B, Groenefeld M, Berg A. 2010 Jul. In Eur J Clin Nutr. ;64(7):762-4.: Glycaemic And Insulinaemic Properties Of Some German Honey Varieties.

[21] Al-Waili NS.. Natural Honey Lowers Plasma Glucose, C-Reactive Protein, Homocysteine, And Blood Lipids In Healthy, Diabetic, And Hyperlipidemic Subjects: Comparison With Dextrose And Sucrose. J Med Food. 2004 Spring;7(1):100-7

[22] A Samanta, Et Al, "Plasma Glucose Responses To Glucose, Sucrose, And Honey In Patients With Diabetes Mellitus: An Analysis Of Glycaemic And Peak Incremental Indices." Diabet Med 1985 Sep; 2(5): 371-373.

[23] Gurung, Manoj & Li, Zhipeng & You, Hannah & Rodrigues, Richard & Jump, Donald & Morgun, Andrey & Shulzhenko, Natalia. (2020). Role of gut microbiota in type 2 diabetes pathophysiology. EBioMedicine. 51. 102590. 10.1016/j.ebiom.2019.11.051.

[24] OO Erejuwa, Et Al, "Honey–A Novel Antidiabetic Agent." Int J Biol Sci 2012; 8(6): 913-34.

[25] GBKS Prasad, Et Al, "Subjects With Impaired Glucose Intolerance Exhibit A High Degree Of Tolerance To Honey." Journal Of Medicinal Food 10(3) 2007: 473-478.

[26] NF Sheard, Et Al, "Dietary Carbohydrate (Amount And Type) In The Prevention And Management Of Diabetes." Diabetes Care 2004; 27:2266-2271.

[27] M Abdulrhman, Et Al, "Effects Of Honey, Sucrose And Glucose On Blood Glucose And C-Peptide In Patients With Type 1 Diabetes Mellitus." Complement Ther Clin Pract 2013 Feb; 19(1): 15-9.

[28] M Abdulrhman, Et Al, "Metabolic Effects Of Honey In Type 1 Diabetes Mellitus: A Randomized Crossover Pilot Study." J Med Food 2013 Jan; 16(1): 66-72.

[29] Münstedt, K; Böhme, M; Hauenschild, A; Hrgovic, I (2011) Consumption Of Rapeseed Honey Leads To Higher Serum Fructose Levels Compared With Analogue Glucose/Fructose Solutions. European Journal Of Clinical Nutrition 65: 77-80.

[30] Meteoglu, Irem & Kavas, Nazli & Saricaoglu, Muge & Ilkaya, Fatih & Guzel, Hasan & ALICI, Omer & Ozturk, Ferhat. (2015). Chestnut Honey And Sherbet Enhance The Healing Of Burn Wounds In Rat Model. Clinical And Investigative Medicine. Médecine Clinique Et Experimentale. 38. 267-273.

[31] Majtán J, Kovácová E, Bíliková K, Simúth J. The Immunostimulatory Effect Of The Recombinant Apalbumin 1-Major Honeybee Royal Jelly Protein-On Tnfalpha Release. Int Immunopharmacol. 2006 Feb;6(2):269-78. Epub (2005 Sep 6).

[32] Bilikova, K; Simuth, J (2010) New Criterion For Evaluation Of Honey: Quantification Of Royal Jelly Protein Apalbumin 1 In Honey By ELISA. Journal Of Agricultural And Food Chemistry 58 (15): 8776-8781.

[33] Małaczewska J, Siwicki AK, Wójcik RM, Kaczorek E, Turski WA. Effect of oral administration of kynurenic acid on the activity of the peripheral blood leukocytes in mice. *Cent Eur J Immunol.* 2014;39(1):6-13. doi:10.5114/ceji.2014.42115

[34] Turski, Michal & Chwil, Stanisław & Turska, Monika & Chwil, Mirosława & Kocki, Tomasz & Rajtar, Grażyna & Parada-Turska, Jolanta. (2016). An Exceptionally High Content Of Kynurenic Acid In Chestnut Honey And Flowers Of Chestnut Tree. Journal Of Food Composition And Analysis. 48. 67-72. 10.1016/J.Jfca.2016.02.003.

[35] Kwakman, P., Te Velde, A., De Boer, L., Speijer, D., Vandenbroucke-Grauls, C., & Zaat, S. (2010). How Honey Kills Bacteria The FASEB Journal, 24 (7), 2576-2582 DOI: 10.1096/Fj.09-150789

[36] Riboulet-Chavey A, Pierron A, Durand I, Murdaca J, Giudicelli J, Van Obberghen E. Methylglyoxal Impairs The Insulin Signaling Pathways Independently Of The Formation Of Intracellular Reactive Oxygen Species. Diabetes. 2006;55(5):1289-1299. Doi:10.2337/Db05-0857

[37] Ron Fessenden, MD- The New Honey Revolution- Kindle E-Book Location: 1245

[38] Meteoglu, Irem & Kavas, Nazli & Saricaoglu, Muge & Ilkaya, Fatih & Guzel, Hasan & ALICI, Omer & Ozturk, Ferhat. (2015). Chestnut Honey And Sherbet Enhance The

Healing Of Burn Wounds In Rat Model. Clinical And Investigative Medicine. Médecine Clinique Et Experimentale. 38. 267-273.

[39] Larson-Meyer DE, Willis KS, Willis LM, et al. Effect of honey versus sucrose on appetite, appetite-regulating hormones, and postmeal thermogenesis. *J Am Coll Nutr.* 2010;29(5):482-493. doi:10.1080/07315724.2010.10719885

40 Samat S, Kanyan Enchang F, Nor Hussein F, Wan Ismail WI. Four-Week Consumption of Malaysian Honey Reduces Excess Weight Gain and Improves Obesity-Related Parameters in High Fat Diet Induced Obese Rats. Evid Based Complement Alternat Med. 2017;2017:1342150. doi:10.1155/2017/1342150

[41] Davis CD. The Gut Microbiome and Its Role in Obesity. *Nutr Today.* 2016;51(4):167-174. doi:10.1097/NT.0000000000000167

[42] HP Rang and MM Dale, Fructose Recycling of NAD from NADH. Pharmacology Churchill Livingstone 1991, Edinburgh Chapter 39, pp 890-891.

PROPOLIS:

[43] Ansorge S, Reinhold D, Lendeckel U. Propolis And Some Of Its Constituents Down-Regulate DNA Synthesis And Inflammatory Cytokine Production But Induce TGF-Beta1 Production Of Human Immune Cells. Z Naturforsch C J Biosci. 2003 Jul-Aug;58(7-8):580-9.

[44] Baltas N1, Karaoglu SA2, Tarakci C2, Kolayli S3 Effect Of Propolis In Gastric Disorders: Inhibition Studies On The Growth Of Helicobacter Pylori And Production Of Its Urease. J Enzyme Inhib Med Chem. 2016;31(Sup2):46-50. Epub 2016 May 27.

[45] Chan GC, Cheung KW, Sze DM The Immunomodulatory And Anticancer Properties Of Propolis. Clin Rev Allergy Immunol. 2013 Jun;44(3):262-73. Doi: 10.1007/S12016-012-8322-2.

[46] Baltas N, Karaoglu SA, Tarakci C, Kolayli S. Effect Of Propolis In Gastric Disorders: Inhibition Studies On The Growth Of Helicobacter Pylori And Production Of Its Urease. J Enzyme Inhib Med Chem. 2016;31(Sup2):46-50. Epub 2016 May 27.

[47] Varanda E.A., Monti R., Tavares D.C. Inhibitory Effect Of Propolis And Bee Venom On The Mutagenicity Of Some Direct- And Indirect-Acting Mutagens. Teratog. Carcinog. Mutagen. 1999;19:403–413. Doi: 10.1002/(SICI)1520-6866(1999)19:6<403::AID-TCM4>3.0.CO;2-2.

[48] Yoon H., Kim M.J., Yoon I., Li D.X., Bae H., Kim S.K. Nicotinic Acetylcholine Receptors Mediate The Suppressive Effect Of An Injection Of Diluted Bee Venom Into The GV3 Acupoint On Oxaliplatin-Induced Neuropathic Cold Allodynia In Rats. Biol. Pharm. Bull. 2015;38:710–714. Doi: 10.1248/Bpb.B14-00797.

[49] Gajski G., Garaj-Vrhovac V. Radioprotective Effects Of Honeybee Venom (Apis Mellifera) Against 915-Mhz Microwave Radiation-Induced DNA Damage In Wistar Rat Lymphocytes: In Vitro Study. Int. J. Toxicol. 2009;28:88–98. Doi: 10.1177/1091581809335051.

[50] Huh J.E., Baek Y.H., Lee M.H., Choi D.Y., Park D.S., Lee J.D. Bee Venom Inhibits Tumor Angiogenesis And Metastasis By Inhibiting Tyrosine Phosphorylation Of VEGFR-2 In LLC-Tumor-Bearing Mice. Cancer Lett. 2010;292:98–110. Doi: 10.1016/J.Canlet.2009.11.013.

[51] Molecules. 2016 May; 21(5): 616. doi: 10.3390/molecules21050616 Anti-Inflammatory Applications of Melittin, a Major Component of Bee Venom: Detailed Mechanism of Action and Adverse Effects, Gihyun Lee and Hyunsu Bae, Derek J. McPhee, Academic Editor

[52] Lee, J.D., Et.Al., (2005) An Overview Of Bee Venom Acupuncture In The Treatment Of Arthritis, Evidence-Based Complementary And Alternative Medicine; 2(1): 79–84.

[53] Lee, J.D., Et.Al., (2005) An Overview Of Bee Venom Acupuncture In The Treatment Of Arthritis, Evidence-Based Complementary And Alternative Medicine; 2(1): 79–84.

[54] James A. Vick, Ben Mehlman, Robert Brooks, Stephen J. Phillips, William Shipman, Effect of bee venom and melittin on plasma cortisol in the unanesthetized monkey, Toxicon, Volume 10, Issue 6, 1972, Pages 581-586, ISSN 0041-0101, https://doi.org/10.1016/0041-0101(72)90119-5.

[55] Lee J.Y., Kang S.S., Kim J.H., Bae C.S., Choi S.H. Inhibitory Effect Of Whole Bee Venom In Adjuvant-Induced Arthritis. In Vivo. 2005;19:801–805.

[56] Son D.J., Lee J.W., Lee Y.H., Song H.S., Lee C.K., Hong J.T. Therapeutic Application Of Anti-Arthritis, Pain-Releasing, And Anti-Cancer Effects Of Bee Venom And Its Constituent Compounds. Pharmacol. Ther. 2007;115:246–270. Doi: 10.1016/J.Pharmthera.2007.04.004.

[57] Tu WC, Wu CC, Hsieh HL, Chen CY, Hsu SL. Honeybee venom induces calcium-dependent but caspase-independent apoptotic cell death in human melanoma A2058 cells. Toxicon. 2008 Aug 1;52(2):318-29. doi: 10.1016/j.toxicon.2008.06.007. Epub 2008 Jun 17. PMID: 18602939.

[58] Vazquez-Revuelta P, Madrigal-Burgaleta R Allergy Division, Ramon Y Cajal University Hospital, Madrid, Spain Death Due To Live Bee Acupuncture Apitherapy, J Investig Allergol Clin Immunol 2018; Ol 28(1) : 45-46 Doi: 10.18176/Jiaci.0202

[59] Eva Sapi [1,*],Rumanah S. Kasliwala [1],Hebo Ismail [1],Jason P. Torres [1],Michael Oldakowski [1],Sarah Markland [1],Gauri Gaur [1],Anthony Melillo [1],Klaus Eisendle [2],Kenneth B. Liegner [3,4,5],Jenny Libien [6] And James E. Goldman [7] The Long-Term Persistence Of Borrelia Burgdorferi Antigens And DNA In The Tissues Of A Patient With Lyme Disease Antibiotics, 2019, 8(4), 183; Https://Doi.Org/10.3390/Antibiotics8040183

[60] Lubke LL [1], Garon CF The Antimicrobial Agent Melittin Exhibits Powerful In Vitro Inhibitory Effects On The Lyme Disease Spirochete. Clin Infect Dis. 1997 Jul;25 Suppl 1:S48-51.

[61] Hood JL, Jallouck AP, Campbell N, Ratner L, Wickline SA. Cytolytic nanoparticles attenuate HIV-1 infectivity. Antiviral Therapy. Vol. 19: 95 – 103. 2013

[62] Wei Yang, Fu-liang Hu, Xiao-feng Xu, Bee venom and SARS-CoV-2, Toxicon, Volume 181, 2020, Pages 69-70, ISSN 0041-0101, https://doi.org/10.1016/j.toxicon.2020.04.105.

[63] Block, Janice. (2020). High risk COVID-19: intervening at multiple points in the COVID-19 disease process via prophylactic treatment with azithromycin or bee derived products. 10.20944/preprints202004.0013.v1.

[64] Kox M, van Eijk LT, Zwaag J, et al. Voluntary activation of the sympathetic nervous system and attenuation of the innate immune response in humans. *Proc Natl Acad Sci U S A*. 2014;111(20):7379-7384. doi:10.1073/pnas.1322174111